AGEING AND THE CRISIS IN HEALTH AND SOCIAL CARE

Global and National Perspectives

Bethany Simmonds

First published in Great Britain in 2022 by

Policy Press, an imprint of
Bristol University Press
University of Bristol
1–9 Old Park Hill
Bristol
BS2 8BB
UK
t: +44 (0)117 954 5940
e: bup-info@bristol.ac.uk

Details of international sales and distribution partners are available at
policy.bristoluniversitypress.co.uk

British Library Cataloguing in Publication Data
A catalogue record for this book is available from the British Library

ISBN 978-1-4473-4859-7 hardcover
ISBN 978-1-4473-4873-3 ePub
ISBN 978-1-4473-4872-6 ePdf

Cover design: Bristol University Press
Front cover image: Wim Lanclus/Alamy
Bristol University Press and Policy Press use environmentally responsible print partners.
Printed by TJ Books, Padstow

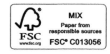

Contents

Acknowledgements

This book is dedicated to all those (older) people who died during the years of austerity policies and the COVID-19 pandemic.

I would like to thank my family and friends for keeping me strong while writing this book, especially when I have suffered multiple health problems over the past three years. Notably, even though I possess 'cultural capital', I now have first-hand experience of the frustrations of navigating health care systems and the postcode lottery of receiving good quality care. Furthermore, during the COVID-19 pandemic, I have been part of the 'shielded' community, providing further insight into the themes of this book.

Most importantly, however, I would like to thank my mentor and the series editor Professor Chris Phillipson for all his encouragement and support; this book would not have been written without it. Thank you to all the supportive colleagues (including those at Policy Press) who have helped me along my journey. There are too many to name here, but you know who you are. Finally, my thanks to the University of Portsmouth for awarding me a Themes Research and Innovation Fund (TRIF) fellowship in 2018, which also supported me in writing this book.

Series editors' preface

Chris Phillipson (University of Manchester, UK)
Toni Calasanti (Virginia Tech, USA)
Thomas Scharf (University of Newcastle, UK)

As the global older population continues to expand, new issues and concerns arise for consideration by academics, policy makers and health and social care professionals worldwide. *Ageing in a Global Context* is a series of books, published by Policy Press in association with the British Society of Gerontology, which aims to influence and transform debates in what has become a fast-moving field in research and policy. The series seeks to achieve this in three main ways: first, through publishing books which re-think the key questions shaping debates in the study of ageing. This has become especially important given the re-structuring of welfare states, alongside the complex nature of population change, both of these elements opening up the need to explore themes which go beyond traditional perspectives in social gerontology. Second, the series represents a response to the impact of globalization and related processes, these contributing to the erosion of the national boundaries which originally framed the study of ageing. From this has come the emergence of issues explored in various contributions to the series, for example: the impact of cultural diversity, changing patterns of working life, new forms of inequality, the role of ethnicity in later life, and related concerns. Third, a key concern of the series is to explore interdisciplinary connections in gerontology. Contributions to the series provide a critical assessment of the disciplinary boundaries and territories influencing later life, creating, in the process, new perspectives and approaches relevant to the 21st century.

Of particular importance has been the crisis in health and social care, driven by changing patterns of ownership and delivery of services, cuts in public spending, and the impact of COVID-19. These changes have themselves interacted with global changes in systems of social protection, these having the effect of introducing new forms of insecurity and precarity. Given this context, Bethany Simmonds provides a significant contribution to the Policy Press/BSG series, illuminating both the impact of neo-liberal policies on older people, but also staff working within the care system. Her study outlines the wider economic and social context in which care is situated, along with valuable case studies of the experiences of older people themselves. The book should prove essential reading for policy makers, practitioners, and academics, working to improve the quality of care and support provided to older people.

Introduction

Contextualising care

Throughout our lives, we all want to give and receive care, particularly at the beginning and the end. The expectation that there will be someone to care for us in later life is almost universal. Women were, and still are, usually tasked with this role, due to what is viewed as their 'naturally' existing caring nature (Hayes, 2017: 80–1). The daily activities of cleaning, cooking, washing and feeding have often been taken for granted and rendered invisible within social structures. Little value has been placed on these life-sustaining tasks (The Care Collective, 2020). Waves of feminism have highlighted the injustices of care work being feminised, devalued and not recognised as 'work' (Hayes, 2017). Yet, women are still providing most of the care for relatives in the family as well as in outside agencies, being paid to provide care services in either domiciliary settings or within residential institutions (Bunting, 2020). Thus, the historical connotations of care work being of low value and feminised have continued. Both formally and informally, women are overwhelmingly those still doing health and social care work with older people (Bunting, 2020). This, coupled with endemic ageism in society (Ayalon and Tesch-Romer, 2018), is arguably how neoliberal governments have successfully justified the low value and pay associated with health and care work, and the low political priority given to the care of older people. In the spring of 2020, the COVID-19 pandemic exposed the years of underfunding, understaffing and privatisation within the sector to devastating effect, as thousands of older people died needlessly in the UK and around the world (The Care Collective, 2020). The care of people with the least power in society mirrors broader political values. As Sevenhuijsen (1998: 4) states:

> The nursing home can be seen as a microcosm of a wider *political* community, in which, as citizens we are continually invited to pass political judgements on the quality of public and private care provision and many different aspects of human social existence.

The treatment of the most vulnerable members of society in this pandemic does not present the UK government in a good light and will hopefully lead to a transformation of health and social care services.

This book illustrates the extent to which global changes in financial and economic systems have undermined care services both in the community and in residential settings. Neoliberal politics in countries in the Global North have deconstructed the social protections afforded to both older people and workers in the post-war era. The changes made to welfare state benefits with respect to pensions, employment regulations, in- and out-of-work benefits, and access to social care services have led to high levels of precarity for both service users and workers alike. Many groups within the older population can no longer retire knowing that they will have a living income, be cared for and not be neglected, without the risk of having to sell their homes or use their life savings to pay for health and social care services. Not all health and social care service workers have welfare policies protecting them against zero-hour contracts, low or frozen pay, exploitation from employers, and unhealthy or risky working conditions. These changes have largely been brought about by sweeping privatisation of the social and health care sector, attributable to a neoliberal agenda under the guise of notions of competition and 'choice'.

The crisis in health and social care is most clearly illustrated when examining older people's experiences and journeys through the health and social care system. The ways in which people attempt to navigate health and social care through its various settings – from public health to pre-emergency care, to hospital and community care – depend on access to resources such as money, family and friends, education, and status. Individuals adept at making informed choices regarding health and social care services, or having relatives that do, will benefit from market competition. This might include buying private health and social care in the form of home adaptations or 24-hour home care services. Fragmented and patchy access to health and social care services has led to greater precarity and inequality among the most vulnerable. This book aims to draw out this layered complexity at the global, national and individual levels, and to demonstrate the impact this has on older people and health care workers.

Setting the scene

I have written this book to provide a critical approach to the social gerontology of health and social care. Firstly, I wanted to demonstrate how neoliberal discourse has shaped economic systems in the Global North through measures such as austerity in the UK. Secondly, the book explores how these neoliberal political discourses have justified the dismantling of social protections for the lowest-paid health and social care workers, while simultaneously undermining the quality of health and social care provision for older people. Thirdly, I examine how these changes to underpinning socio-economic structures have led to privatisation, marketisation and fragmentation of the health and social care sector. Health and social care workers, alongside older people, have suffered significantly under these austerity measures, becoming more vulnerable and experiencing more precarity in their everyday and working lives than ever before. These sufferings were starkly illuminated during the COVID-19 pandemic, which was developing while I was writing this book.

However, the economic crisis of 2008 occurred a year after I began my doctoral research, thus while completing my thesis, I was witnessing a shift in policy emphasis from preventative health located within an active ageing paradigm to austerity policy linked to precarious ageing. The precarity of ageing was then evident in my role as a professional researcher when I worked on multiple projects that involved examining older people's experiences through various pathways of care. Nevertheless, the first care setting I examined as a doctoral student between 2007 and 2011 was public health. I was tasked with looking at the barriers and benefits to older people participating in physical activity. As someone outside the health care profession, this seemed like a reasonably straightforward proposal: find out why many older people are not being physically active and how those that do participate in physical activity benefit from it. However, the assumptions inherent in these questions soon became clear. Why *should* older people be physically active? Do older people feel physical activity is of benefit? What enhances older people's wellbeing in later life? Quickly, the focus of my thesis changed to a critical examination of the neoliberal agenda of imposing active ageing frameworks on older populations in the Global North. I used social theory to examine how discourses of public health shape older people's subjectivities and how these discourses operate through institutions such as the National Health Service (NHS) and other third-sector (those not private or public) organisations, like the British Heart Foundation. Finally, I examined how these public health messages, mediated through institutions, were internalised and embodied, or resisted by older people themselves. This book presents some of the findings of my thesis and applies the same critical analysis to the other health and social care settings from my postdoctoral work.

The second health and social care setting discussed in this book is pre-emergency care, where I worked as a research fellow running a feasibility study between 2013 and 2014 to see whether paramedics attending to older people who had fallen could identify whether they were at risk of low-impact fractures by asking a short series of questions to assess a person's risk of fracturing a bone (known as a FRAX questionnaire). In this role, I shadowed paramedics attending to older people who had fallen, in order to evaluate whether it would be feasible for the paramedics to complete a FRAX questionnaire in such instances/contexts. When I was riding around in the back of the ambulance, I noticed how skilled the paramedics' jobs had become; not only did they transfer patients to hospital, but they also used clinical decision-making skills in assessing, treating and triaging patients to community care by contacting General Practitioners (GPs), social workers, care staff and family members. They found it difficult to negotiate the myriad of services in a fragmented health and social care system. Older patients and their carers, who were supposed to be making informed 'choices' about their current and ongoing care, also struggled to understand and make decisions, especially in pre-emergency settings.

Hospital and community care are the last two health settings discussed in this book. This section draws upon my previously published research from 2012 to 2020, examining the clinical decision-making of senior staff in hospitals when an older person approaches the end of their life and evaluates end of life care services based in the community. Older patients navigating health and social care services at the end of their lives faced similar but slightly different challenges to those being discharged from hospital. On top of the complexity, fragmentation, duplication and inefficiency involved in discharging older patients, there was the stigma and taboo surrounding death. No professional wanted to be responsible for these discussions; GPs were reluctant and clinicians have been trained within the ethos of doing everything to save lives, not to withdraw treatment. Clinicians in emergency care environments were also incredibly busy. To have sensitive, in-depth conversations about end of life in an emergency room setting was challenging to say the least.

When a hospital clinician is able to have a conversation with a dying patient about limiting interventions and that patient is subsequently discharged into the community, the services available to them are inconsistent. Often end of life care hospices are delivered by the third sector, in which palliative care and hospice services vary dramatically, and it is a postcode lottery as to whether older people experience a 'good death'. The challenges of providing sensitive end of life care, and the hospital discharge of older people, were illuminated during the COVID-19 pandemic and are discussed in this book, along with the role public health information plays in taking a preventative approach to health inequalities in later life.

Key takeaways

This book fits between several established fields, including health and social care, ageing and the welfare state, and the sociology of neoliberalism and globalisation. Instead of focusing on one discrete area, the book provides a critical sociological study of austerity politics, and health and social care models in Europe, alongside key contemporary issues, such as the COVID-19 pandemic and Brexit. It also discusses some innovative yet practical solutions to the 'crisis'. It also develops the work of Grenier et al (2020b) on precarity and ageing, which explores themes of globalisation, neoliberalism and declining social protections. This book, however, applies these concepts to the health and social care systems in three countries in the Global North, and analyses the impact of these global and national influences on individuals' experiences of the UK health and social care system. It offers global-, national- and individual-level analyses, discussing the impact of discursive and structural change on health and social care workers and older people.

This book is relevant to several audiences, including sociologists interested in health and social care and ageing, as well as academics, policymakers and commissioners looking for a pragmatic text that suggests potential solutions to the complex issues discussed. Furthermore, practitioners in health and social care will find the individual accounts of older people's care familiar and perhaps resonant with their own experiences, and the book will hopefully provide them with a more theoretical insight into how global and national discourses and structures are shaping these experiences. In this respect, the book contributes to rethinking health and social care in the UK, away from privatisation, marketisation, competition and neoliberal modes of thinking. The case studies of the health and social care systems in Sweden and Germany allow for comparisons with the UK model, highlighting how the neoliberalisation of health and social care services has exceptions in its various forms. Furthermore, the book discusses other innovative schemes and solutions that have been tried in the UK which deserve (re)consideration, particularly following the COVID-19 pandemic.

This book could also interest scholars examining social class and inequality across the lifecourse, as it provides accounts of workers and older people's experiences of a market-based health and social care system that favours those with educational, economic and social capital. Other health care studies have demonstrated that the introduction of choice has not advantaged the groups it was supposed to empower: the working classes. Instead, older people who are working-class and have accumulated disadvantages over the lifecourse find 'choosing' the best care without adequate resources and support particularly difficult.

This book is intended for an international readership, as it examines health and social care in two other European countries (Germany and Sweden) and also discusses the influence of global trends in finance systems, such as neoliberalism and marketisation, which have repercussions throughout the world. Therefore, this book provides readers from countries where health and social care has not yet been privatised with an insight into how the provision of health and social care could look in their countries in the future, and how to prevent the sort of 'crisis' the UK is facing. Furthermore, for readers from countries with similar demographics, such as the US, Canada, Australia, New Zealand, Ireland and Japan, these themes and issues will have more direct applicability. This book will hopefully help the generally interested reader to envisage alternative health and social care possibilities in later life.

Outline of the book

In Chapters 2, 3 and 4, the theoretical and conceptual frameworks of the book will be discussed. Chapter 2, 'Discourse, capital, intersectionality and precarity', lays the theoretical groundwork for the book. In this chapter, I begin by presenting an analysis of neoliberal discourse and how this has shaped global and national health and social care policies by subtly shifting the responsibility of paying for care from the state to the individual. The biopolitical nature of this subtle shift in health responsibilities, driven by the rhetoric of choice, has paved the way for the marketisation of health and social care systems in most countries in the Global North. The dominant theorisations of ageing – biomedical, social-gerontological and 'successful ageing' – are then discussed. The chapter will then go on to discuss the Bourdieusian concepts of capital and field, applying these to the health and social care context. Following this, I discuss how a feminist intersectional analysis, which situates social class alongside other identities (such as age, gender, ethnicity and disability), is important for understanding the heterogeneity of older people. The layering of different identities impacts the levels of inequality older people experience and their ability to access health and social care services.

Chapter 3, 'Globalisation, neoliberalism and welfare state models: a comparative analysis', provides global perspectives on the crisis in health and social care for older people, examining the broad socio-economic structural changes that have occurred in societies in the Global North, particularly with respect to neoliberalism and globalisation, and the effect these have had on health and social care models in countries in the Global North. The chapter provides case study analyses of health and social care policies in Germany and Sweden in order to provide comparisons with those of the UK. In this chapter, the UK, Germany and Sweden are used as exemplifying countries to demonstrate how three archetypal welfare state systems have been affected by neoliberalism, and the resulting privatisation of health and social care services. Prior to a discussion of these two case studies, I examine the impact of globalisation and neoliberalism on privatisation and financing of health and social care in the UK.

Chapter 4, 'Failing health and social care in the UK: austerity, neoliberal ideology and precarity', is the last of the chapters discussing broad discursive and structural trends. This chapter continues with a national-level analysis, examining the impact of globalisation and neoliberalism on health and social care policy in the UK. It starts with a discussion of austerity policy and the ensuing erosion of social protections in relation to employment and working rights of health and social care staff. This is followed by an analysis of the effects of large, private shareholding organisations entering the (low-risk and high-yield) social care market. The conglomerates Southern Cross and Four

Seasons are used as case studies, illustrating how asset-stripping, reductions in labour costs and the weakening of employment law have led to greater precarity for health and social care workers as well as older people.

Chapter 5, 'Public health, emergency settings and end of life care', explores individual-level data related to three health care settings, beginning with public or preventative health. This setting is examined through a discussion of 'active ageing' frameworks, which encourage older people to participate in physical activity. I argue here that neoliberal governments have promoted active ageing frameworks without considering how levels of capital impact older people's ability to participate in physically active lifestyles. I also examine the unintended consequences that arise for those who cannot partake in such lifestyles. The chapter then moves on to the sphere of pre-emergency care, examining a care pathway that older people commonly experience: falling and being attended to by an ambulance. This section reflects on paramedics' experiences of working as frontline health workers in a challenging environment, as well as the experiences of older people, who often end up being left waiting on the floor for several hours after a fall. Finally, this chapter examines end of life care, where I discuss the problems caused by a lack of trained senior clinicians who can make end of life care decisions. The lack of dedicated time and an appropriate environment in which to have these sensitive discussions is also highlighted as a challenge. Like community care services, end of life care is complex and patchy. The services accessible to an older person who is approaching the end of their life is dependent on where they live, whether they have friends or family supporting them, and which clinician is treating them. Being discharged to one's home with the right end of life care and support requires patients to negotiate many factors outside of their control. This is particularly hard to do when someone is at the most precarious and vulnerable phase of their life.

Chapter 6, 'The COVID-19 health and social care challenge', provides an overview of the devastating effects of the COVID-19 pandemic, providing an initial discussion of what went wrong. This is followed by an examination of the COVID-19–Brexit nexus and its impact on health and social care, and the possible ways forward the government may take to solve the multiple crises the UK faces. This includes examining the Conservative government's proposed reconfigurations, including the introduction of 'integrative care systems'. Finally, a comparative analysis of health and social care policies related to COVID-19 in Sweden and Germany will be outlined, revisiting the two case studies detailed in Chapter 4, where Germany and Sweden's health and social care systems were examined. This discussion focuses on what the UK can learn from these countries' responses to the COVID-19 pandemic.

Chapter 7, 'Innovative solutions and cultural change', will discuss innovative alternative health and social care solutions that have undergone trials in the UK but have not been adopted fully. The Homeshare scheme, for example, matches older people who have a spare room with younger people who provide befriending and informal 'care'. As I discuss, there seems to be a cultural dimension as to why this scheme has not been adopted more widely. For instance, cultural questions as to whether it is socially acceptable for non-family members to live together have arisen in relation to this scheme. These questions could reflect something significant about the norms within British culture. This closing chapter emphasises the importance of holistic rather than process–driven solutions, as well as the importance of valuing interdependence over and above independence. Finally, I consider how the COVID-19 pandemic could be a unique opportunity for transformation and change.

2

Discourse, capital, intersectionality and precarity

Introduction

This chapter outlines the theoretical lenses used to frame and discuss the book's themes. Framing discussion using theory is important because it lifts analysis beyond a descriptive account to a more critical examination of how societal structures and discursive developments have impacted institutions. For example, neoliberal and austerity discourse has shaped health and social care structures and institutions, such as the NHS, which have changed the experiences of individuals, such as older people and health or social care workers. Furthermore, it is important to discuss theoretical concepts such as neoliberalism, capital and precarity, in order to illustrate how broad discursive and structural change has influenced levels of security and stability for older people and staff in health and social care. For example, neoliberal discourse, which supports austerity measures and public funding cuts, impacts the resources or capital available to service users and those working in the public sector by making their lives more precarious. The extent to which older people are affected relates to their level of capital (economic, physical, social and cultural [Bourdieu, 1984; Dumas and Turner, 2006]); for example, being more educated or wealthy mediates an older person's access to health and social care systems. Family and friends (social and cultural capital) are particularly important in helping older people traverse and negotiate the complexities of fragmented health and social care services. However, class is not the only identity that can impact older people's access to health care resources. Social class intersects with other identities such as age, gender, disability and ethnicity (Corus and Saatcioglu, 2015). These identity combinations influence access to health and social care, either by layering disadvantages or advantages through one's lifecourse. This chapter will draw on ideas from Michel Foucault (1972) to demonstrate how these identity combinations have shaped older people's access to necessary health resources. Foucauldian theory is being used here to provide a critical lens through which to analyse how and why particular arguments about desired health behaviours have been constructed. Foucault was interested in how language, practice and perceptions shape the world; for instance, he was interested in how some groups, but not others, are enabled to exercise the power to produce knowledge (Foucault, 1972).

Neoliberal health and social care policy discourse: a Foucauldian analysis

Foucault was a philosopher whose writings covered a range of diverse topics including madness, medicine, sexuality and penalty. What linked these topics was their connection to issues of social order and power. Foucault focussed on the conditions and circumstances that enable some groups and not others to make claims that come to be regarded as truth (Turner, 2008). Although Foucault never addressed ageing per se, his work has influenced several writers in gerontology and sociology (see, for example, Katz, 1996, 2005, 2018; Powell and Wahidin, 2006). For instance, Foucault's theories and concepts have been useful when examining ageing, particularly when performing macro analyses of how discourses of ageing shape truths about later life – for example, how a biomedical discourse has dominated ageing narratives, including 'successful ageing' discourses (Simmonds, 2011). His theories have been particularly pertinent to analyses of power relations between groups of 'experts', as although medical professionals have traditionally held the power of truth in relation to older people's health, more recently, social gerontologists have challenged this power base by arguing for a broader and more holistic conceptualisation of ageing.

Foucault (1972) argues that scientific discourses are historically and culturally constructed through networks of power present at different historical times and places. Therefore, ageing discourse is fluid and constantly shifting. The networks of power which are temporally and spatially present restrict and enable certain scientific knowledge frameworks to form, which go on to shape institutions (such as the NHS) (Foucault, 1978, 1991). Foucault (1978) theorised that political 'disciplines', such as demography (which observed birth rates and longevity), emerged in response to the industrial revolution and rapid urban population growth. The state became concerned about the health of the population in these new environments where people lived in close proximity and the impact this would have on their productivity in a capitalist system (Turner, 2008). Therefore, new institutions like the NHS were created to ensure the health of populations, such as workers, mothers of the next generation of workers, and the military who protect the nation–state (Turner, 2008). Therefore, these new fields, like demography, attempt to control populations or the 'social body', by examining birth weights, life expectancy, and levels of chronic illness; this data is used to improve productivity by restricting temporal or spatial activities deemed undesirable to the state (Turner, 2008).

Katz (1996) applied Foucault's theory to ageing and explored the ways in which disciplinary practices and discourses have affected the older social and individual body. For instance, he examined how the discourses surrounding pensions constructed older people as 'needy, dependent and unproductive' (Katz, 1996: 67). In response to these negative discourses of inevitable degeneration and dependency, positive (or 'successful') ageing discourses were created to counteract and resist ageism in society (Levi et al, 2018). However, these discourses have had the unintended consequence of creating binary moral subject positions that serve to reproduce inequalities such as age, social class and gender (Liang and Luo, 2012; Calasanti, 2015). For example, older people who do not have the physical or material resources to inhabit a 'successful ageing' subject position are considered unsuccessful and linked to the 'failed' 'fourth age', rather than the positively connoted 'third age', which is linked to increased leisure time and wellbeing (Higgs and Gilleard, 2014). Arguably, neoliberals have appropriated 'positive' and 'successful ageing' narratives as part of a healthism agenda, which shifts responsibility for one's health from the state onto the individual (Crawford, 1980; Simmonds, 2011).

This shift in expectation that the individual, not the state, should address health and social care needs, has helped to legitimise neoliberal austerity policies. Marmot et al (2020) discuss how austerity policy has led to cuts to local authority funding in the UK, leading to the rationing of social care for older people, which leaves vulnerable individuals responsible for maintaining their own care needs (discussed further in Chapters 3 and 4). However, older people with access to resources are less likely to need health and social care services and are more likely to be White middle-class men who are still active, and those less likely to age successfully are minority ethnic women from working-class backgrounds with lower mobility levels. Discourses of ageing that label older people as 'successful' or 'unsuccessful' according to narrow biomedical measures construct hierarchies of ageing. Older people are placed into aged, gendered and racialised hierarchical subject positions that are 'marked' and problematised (Krekula and Johansson, 2016). Additionally, these hierarchies denote their relative accumulation of cultural and social capital (Bourdieu, 1984). Therefore, discourses of ageing, such as decline and degeneration or successful/positive ageing, impact institutions such as health services, shaping understandings, attitudes, practices and behaviours towards older people (Wyman et al, 2018).

Governmentality and biopolitics

Another useful Foucauldian concept in analysing health and social care policy is 'governmentality', which loosely refers to the ways in which systems of thought operate to govern and respond to social 'problems' using taken-for-granted regimes of practice (Dean, 2010). Foucault identified two main types of governmentality: sovereign and biopolitical (Dean, 2013). In *Discipline and Punish* (1991), Foucault describes sovereign power with vivid imagery of the gallows, dismemberment, torture and brandings in public. The sovereign terrorises their subjects and has ultimate control over punishment if their laws are disobeyed. Biopolitics, in contrast, is conceptualised as a different form of governmental power that is subtler and more insidious (Foucault, 1978). Biopower is a modern form of power, which involves the state governing collectives of individuals via disciplinary practices, through institutions such as the prison, the school, the family and the welfare state (Dean, 2013). However, unlike disciplinary practices that just work on the individual body, biopower regulates whole populations (Dean, 2013) – for example, public health campaigns that target older populations (Hepworth, 1995; Lupton, 1995; Nettleton and Bunton, 2005). Unlike disciplinary power, which uses norms to place judgement on individuals, defining them as 'normal' or 'abnormal', biopower uses statistical data to establish normality (Dean, 2013).

Foucault goes on to argue that biopolitics sits within the larger governmental political framework and mentality of liberalism (Foucault, 2008). When biopolitics, with an overwhelming imperative to sustain life, meets liberalism, a political persuasion concerned with the optimal and most cost-effective method to reach its means, neoliberal methods of free enterprise are produced (Hardin, 2014). Therefore, Foucault indicates that biopolitical governmentality is an ideal method of regulation for liberalism, as it avoids the use of sovereign power, which explicitly defends and promotes state interests; instead, it works through civil society, the population and, most importantly, the economy, using the notion of choice as a technique to exert domination (Dean, 2013). This liberalism is of course not political liberalism (based on the principles of laissez-faire), but a particular kind of economic liberalism linked to 'state phobia', and an early form of neoliberalism which emerged first in Germany and then later in the United States (Foucault, 2008). The nature of this state-phobia is a repulsion against John Maynard Keynes' notion of economic intervention and planning of the economy. Thus, this form of liberalism legitimises and justifies state intervention, the regulation of the market economy and creating a society constructed on the principle of competition. Therefore, if the very legitimacy of the state is based on the market, this justifies strategies that construct and support the economy via economic trade and taxation policies, but also via complementary social policies that ensure that risk is individualised. This justifies a realm of possible interventions (Foucault, 2008), from legislating that a large percentage of social care is provided by the private sector in the UK (see Chapter 3), to the British government COVID-19 policy which recommended individuals 'stay alert' against the risk of infection (see Chapter 6).

Biomedical theorisation of ageing

The dualistic Cartesian theorisation of separating the mind and the body is ubiquitous to Western thought and is especially dominant in biomedical approaches to ageing (Tulle, 2015). For example, notions of healthy ageing which have separated the 'active mind' and the 'busy body' (Paulson and Willig, 2008) are endemic in ageing narratives. This detachment of mind and body can be located within a decline discourse, as to do so acts to distance and distract the individual from their ageing body (Katz, 2000). Since the industrial revolution, this dualistic biomedical theorisation has been extended to machinery, proposing that ageing bodies 'wear and tear' or behave according to in-built programming which over time, 'turns off' (Allesio, 1999, cited in Powell et al, 2006: 9). The inevitable decline and biological determinism implicit in this theorisation have been criticised for ignoring the many social, cultural and technological factors that restrict older people when trying to achieve a full and active life (Estes and Binney, 1989; Twigg and Martin, 2015).

In the wake of modernity, older bodies and older populations became central to biopolitics (Katz, 2000). Biomedical discourse dominated social knowledge and, as previously discussed, was used to shape the economic efficiency of the workforce. According to Foucault (1978), concepts of illness and disease have become part of a wider structure, controlling and regulating vulnerable groups in society. As Powell and Wahidin (2006: viii) note, 'Foucault has problematized the role of the "expert", social institutions, social processes and subjectivity that seem "empowering" but are contingent socio-historical constructions and products of power and domination'. Neoliberal governments have used knowledge collected by 'experts' such as doctors, to design interventions that aim to maintain and reproduce age-related power relations (Powell and Wahidin, 2006).

Ageing is still largely understood as being synonymous with illness and disease (Gilleard, 2018), and the subject of biomedical interventions such as hormone-replacement therapy to treat menopause (Turner, 2000). As a result of public health policies in the Global North, women's bodies in particular have been subject to scrutiny of their physical attractiveness and evaluation of their propensity for harm using biomedicalised notions of risk and beauty (Calasanti, 2020a). This medicalisation of older populations has increased in intensity, with more healthy populations being defined as 'at risk', which has continued to legitimise increased surveillance (Powell et al, 2006).

Biomedical conceptualisations of risk have been particularly influential in relation to falls in later life, with individual and health costs cited to justify this focus (Katz, 2000). Positivist approaches that record and attempt to minimise risk have worked to disassociate health care professionals' understandings of falls from the social context and have discouraged the independent movement of older people (Ballanger and Payne, 2002). In contrast, older people's perceptions of risk in later life are centred on the threat falling poses to their sense of self and identity; for example, being labelled 'a faller' can be experienced as 'infantilising' (Ballanger and Payne, 2002). Therefore, biomedical narratives are controversial in often failing to consider the social context or subjective experience of later life. Further, they encourage the construction of binary categories, such as functional/dysfunctional and normal/abnormal, into which the corporeal status of older people are placed. Moreover, through this categorisation and labelling of ageing bodies with age-related stereotypes, social and economic marginalisation is reproduced (Krekula et al, 2018).

Social-gerontological theories of ageing

Social-gerontological approaches to ageing in the 1960s were critiqued by Estes (1979), among others, for constructing a dependency narrative, suggesting that older people should or need to be dependent on the state. For example, disengagement theory, based on a functionalist understanding of efficiency and the division of labour, proposed that ageing is a natural and inevitable process of withdrawal from society into retirement, which is beneficial for both society and the individual (Turner, 1987). Disengagement theory failed to acknowledge individual differences and the possibility that withdrawal from society for some older people is unwanted and detrimental to their wellbeing. Critique of these theories drew attention to the lack of acknowledgement that older people may not be able to withdraw into a comfortable and satisfying retirement (Turner, 1987). Moreover, disengagement theory combines an economically deterministic understanding of ageing, which reduces older people's value to their economic productivity, with a biomedical reductionist understanding. This results in ageing being understood as a process of inevitable decline and dependency on the state.

In the 1970s and '80s, writers such as Estes (1979), Townsend (1981) and Myles (1984) questioned the assumption of 'natural withdrawal' and argued instead that dependency is socially constructed through retirement policies, marginalisation, poverty and institutionalisation (Walker, 1981; Townsend, 1981). These political-economic approaches argued that dependency discourses disregard older people's (former) identities, contributions and legitimate segregationist welfare policies (Phillipson 1998). This critique of the dependency narrative, however, has also been criticised for being overly structurally deterministic in suggesting that older people have little agency in resisting the state (Phillipson, 1998). However, since the onset of neoliberal politics in the 1980s, the discussion has shifted from dependence per se to deservedness (Calasanti, 2020a). The most economically vulnerable have been classified as 'burdens' and, in the case of older people, this has been constructed with the aid of dependency ratios (Calasanti, 2020a). Crude dependency ratios leave out younger people who are fully economically dependent on the working population; this omission skews the statistics and when included demonstrates a total dependency ratio that does not show a dramatic increase over time (Macnicol, 2015). Furthermore, contrary to media discourse, older people are productive in society providing various forms of unpaid work, including caring responsibilities (Lain, 2018) and sharing their life experiences in voluntary settings (Calasanti, 2020a). These contributions are conveniently overlooked in neoliberal discourse, which constructs older people's pensions or health and social care costs as being in competition with public provision for younger people, with the latter being more deserving of investment (Calasanti, 2020a; see Chapter 6 for discussion of 'new ageism'). Thus, although critiques of discourse constructing older people as dependent are well-rehearsed, they still have to be vocalised when zero-sum arguments regarding resource rationing are operationalised.

Successful/active ageing theory

Although various incarnations of ageing counter-narratives (e.g. 'successful', 'active', 'positive', 'healthy' and 'productive' ageing) have been used interchangeably, in social gerontology, 'active ageing' is understood in policy terms (Lassen and Moirera, 2014) whereas 'successful ageing' is more conceptual (Liang and Luo, 2012). For instance, Timonen (2016: 35) explains the connection between the concept of successful ageing and active ageing models: 'Gerontologists have contributed to the translation of successful ageing ideation into the policy sphere, where ideas take on more practice-orientated form; this is a manifestation of what I call modelling ageing.' Nonetheless, the successful ageing concept is not new and its origins can be found in Havighurst's (1961) activity theory, which was also developed as a critique of disengagement theory (Cumming and Henry, 1961). The concept was an attempt to provide an alternative, more positive, ageing narrative, which advocated for older people's active engagement in social activities to replace those provided by work (Timonen, 2016). Successful ageing has subsequently been operationalised both subjectively and objectively (Rowe and Kahn, 1987). What has been more dominant is propagating that successful ageing can be objectively identified and that successful outcomes can be overwhelmingly controlled by older people themselves via their lifestyle choices (Timonen, 2016). In so doing, conceptualisations of successful ageing have also been medicalised and removed from their social contexts; subjective experiences of what it means to older people to age successfully have been ignored, particularly in reference to diverse cultural, ethnic and classed identities (Katz and Calasanti, 2015). Thus, notions of 'success' in later life have been divorced from culturally and temporally defined conceptualisations of what it means to be older (Wray, 2003, 2004).

In policy terms, successful ageing seems to have translated well into active ageing frameworks (Timonen, 2016). Like successful ageing, active ageing has become a broad umbrella response to all demographic developments (Walker and Foster, 2013). Active ageing policy frameworks have proliferated since 2002, when the World Health Organization (WHO) started to promote policies that included older people in society (WHO, 2002). The WHO's framework for active ageing – 'the process of optimising opportunities for health, participation and security in order to enhance the quality of life as people age' (WHO, 2002: 12) – has shaped the policy frameworks of national-level institutions such as the Research Councils UK (2009) and the Department of Health (DH, 2011). While the WHO's original active ageing framework projected a holistic understanding of health and wellbeing, physical activity has become a central focus of these national efforts in the UK (Grant, 2002). In other European countries, however, a more flexible 'lifecourse' policy approach to the challenges of ageing has been operationalised. As Walker and Foster (2013) argue, there are two interpretations of active ageing policy: one is economically reductionist and the other is holistic and subjective. Nevertheless, the one operationalised by national and international organisations is usually the former: narrowly interpreted and focused on physical activity. Therefore, there is no inclusion within active or successful ageing narratives of fourth-age experiences of decline and degeneration. Instead, the fourth-age subject position is characterised with all unwelcome ageing attributes (Higgs and Gilleard, 2015). According to Laslett's seminal work (1989), the third age is characterised as a life stage where physical activity and active engagement in social networks take place; the fourth age is characterised by dependency and decline. As these are undesirable characteristics in a neoliberal state, UK governments have used preventative health policies, such as those promoted via active/healthy/positive ageing frameworks, to minimise the financial implications of later life and distract discussion away from the structural inequalities shaping individuals' health (Simmonds, 2011).

Bourdieusian theory applied to ageing

Although Bourdieu did not theorise or discuss ageing, his work is uniquely suited to understanding class distinctions in later life (Gilleard, 2020). Capitals capture the heterogeneity of material and symbolic statuses of older people in society (Gilleard, 2020). Bourdieu's (1984) concept of the field refers to an 'arena of production', or a space where individuals invest and compete for resources. Within these fields or social spaces, individuals can exert different levels of power based on their possession of a variety of different resources

(Bourdieu, 1984). These powerful resources, or 'capital', come in different forms: cultural, symbolic and social (Bourdieu, 1984). *Cultural capital* refers to the power people accumulate through education and family background (Laberge and Kay, 2002). *Symbolic capital* refers to the individual's legitimate demand for social recognition (Laberge and Kay, 2002). *Social capital* refers to resources based on social connections and membership of social groups (Bourdieu, 1977, 1987). Furthermore, Camerer and Hogarth (1999) have applied Bourdieu's theorisation of capital to labour theory to encapsulate the power that knowledge provides individuals when consuming services or products in a market, known as *cognitive capital*. This theorisation is useful when examining older people's ability to make choices in the consumption of health and social care. Finally, Dumas and Turner (2006) also apply Bourdieu's concept of capital to the ageing body in order to develop the concept of *physical capital*, referring to the loss of corporeal aesthetic, strength, vitality and, ultimately, power. As a result of different levels of capital and lifestyles, individuals, according to Bourdieu (1984), are hierarchically situated in social space; those with the most capital are situated at the top of the hierarchy while those at the bottom have the least access to power.

This is no difference in the field of health and social care. Patients use their educational, social and economic capital to obtain the best services and health outcomes they can. The effect of levels of capital is particularly pertinent for older people, who use and need national health care services proportionately more than younger people. There are other reasons why, as a group, older people have particular experiences of health and social care services. When people reach the fourth age, they tend to share some common physical experiences, including aches, pains and tiredness. Dumas and Turner (2006) termed this 'ageing habitus', which describes how corporeal experiences shape individuals' interactions with the outside world. These experiences in turn change an individual's sense of self. They become labelled and treated as an 'older person' by society, changing their everyday movements according to this new aged identity. Like any other social space, this identity construction is also true within the field of health.

Older people who hold low levels of symbolic capital (in relation to classed, gendered, abled and ethnic status) are also less likely to have accumulated economic capital throughout their lifecourses. Healthy life expectancy is shorter for individuals who live in more deprived areas (Marmot et al, 2020). Subsequently, when poorer people do fall ill, they are not ideally located to be able to navigate the health and social care system, as they experience more barriers than those holding more symbolic capital. The influence of family members acting as advocates for more fortunate older people has a significant positive effect on their navigation through various patient pathways in the fields of community, emergency, secondary and primary care. Families and communities can provide support to prevent a decline in health, advocate on the older person's behalf in an emergency and provide support in secondary care with treatment and discharge. They can also minimise the risk of the older person being readmitted once discharged from secondary care by ensuring that they have the right equipment, food, transport and access to community services.

In summary, the value attributed to older people in society is shaped by theories of ageing which contribute to the prevalence of ageism, the denigration of ageing bodies and, ultimately, a preoccupation with sequestering and delaying death. As a result, older people hold less symbolic capital in the health care system than younger people. This is also the case for other identities, such as class, gender and ethnicity. Those holding lower symbolic capital, for instance, older, minority ethnic, working-class women, would be those most precarious in this field.

Intersections of age, gender, disability and ethnicity

Intersectional theory originates from a Black feminist critique of deterministic and ethnocentric feminist theory, problematising assumptions of universality (Crenshaw, 1989). Women's experiences are stratified by a multitude of other identities, such as social class, ethnicity, age and disability. These identities impact the experiences of older women in the health and social care system. Although strictly more of an additive than an intersectional theorisation, Chappell and Havens (1980) describe the combination of age and gender inequalities as a form of 'double jeopardy'. Older women are exposed to double the discrimination: as women age, they are losing not only their productive value in a capitalist system, but also their sexual value. In the Global North, menopause is synonymous with denigration and decline; it is medicalised as a disease, instead of being celebrated as a part of a woman's lifecourse. Thus, menopause is conceptualised as a loss of womanhood and the sexual function of a woman's body: a border crossing symbolising a shift from a fertile productive woman to a diseased, desexualised being (Adkins and Holland, 1996). The media is particularly influential in constructing and policing this shift, with women's appearance relentlessly scrutinised for signs of ageing. Plastic surgery, makeup, fitness regimes and body modifications are normalised in Western culture (Shilling, 2003). Women in the media are particularly under pressure to mould and shape their bodies to society's expectations for them to be ageless (Pike, 2010). Thus, older women tend to experience both discrimination for being a woman and for being older – a double whammy (Arber and Ginn, 1998). The combination of these two identities is transposed into the health and social care system. Furthermore, issues of body modification also intersect with classed identities.

Women from middle-class backgrounds not only have had access to more cultural capital throughout their lifetime (e.g. in the form of formal and informal education), but also to economic capital, which they can use to shape, nip and tuck their bodies into a desired corporeal identity and to remain youthful. Middle-class women have greater access to health services throughout their lifetime, but also have access to 'healthier' lifestyles that incorporate physical activities such as yoga or going to the gym (Parviainen, 2001). Furthermore, middle-class women are more likely to live in environments with less pollution, to have occupations that carry less risk to health and to not have worked in manual jobs, increasing their availability for leisure (Dumas and Laberge, 2005).

Extending Chappell and Havens' analysis, Norman (1985) uses the term 'triple jeopardy' to highlight the specific challenges that older people from minority ethnic backgrounds have when accessing health care services. For instance, language, cultural and economic barriers can be seen to play an important part in preventing access to health and social care services. The intersections of ethnicity and class are well known as playing key mediating roles in the field of health (Graham, 2009). Whether in relation to housing, employment, environmental pollution, education or money, people from minority ethnic backgrounds are likely to possess less capital than their White counterparts, and they are more likely to be working-class.

Finally, some of the literature on ageing and disability overlaps and the two concepts have sometimes been conflated. However, age and disability are two distinctive identities. For instance, those who have become 'dis'abled earlier in life have very different experiences and needs to those individuals who have become 'dis'abled as they have aged (Lowton and Higgs, 2010). Yet, research on disabled people's experiences highlights some similar embodied experiences of accessing health and social care to those of older people (Thomas, 2007). Impairment models imply a continuum of ability; they argue that to some extent everyone has some sort of impairment (Thomas, 2007). Further, in this model, the lived corporeal experience of 'dis'ability is explored; for example, whether someone was born with a hearing impairment or they acquired it in later life will have an impact on their experience (Thomas, 2007). For health and social care interactions, impairments result in a reduction of physical capital, a propensity to be a regular health care user and to be more precarious economically due to the discrimination against 'dis'abled or impaired people within the workforce (Dixton et al, 2018). Thus, impairment and disability also form a layer of inequality when older people access health and social care services.

Arguably, when class, ethnicity, 'dis'ability and age are combined with gender, a quintuple jeopardy is formed. As previously stated, older, minority ethnic, 'dis'abled, working-class women tend to be the most precariously placed within the health and social care system. This is also the case for workers in the health and social care system; those who have layers of identities that lead to multiple inequalities and precarity are often women from minority ethnic communities, the working classes and those with impairments themselves (see Chapter 6 for a discussion of the impact of COVID-19).

Theorising precarity and ageing

The concept of precarity has many different interpretations and applications across several disciplines, but it has most commonly been applied to the examination of working practices and policy in relation to employees rather than to service users (such as older people). The general meaning of precarity relates to people's risky positionings in the socio-economic system, although there are substantive variations that will be outlined in the following sections. So far, there has been little research on older people's precarious positioning in relation to the radical changes in global and national policies and practices as a result of globalisation, neoliberalism and austerity.

There is an extensive field of literature in labour studies in relation to precarity (Grenier et al, 2020b). For example, Campbell and Price (2016) have examined how notions of precariousness, precarious work and precarious workers are often blurred. For clarity, they conceptualised precariousness in five levels; 'precarious employment', 'precarious work', 'precarious workers', 'precariat' and 'precarity'. 'Precarious employment' refers to the characteristics of a job that lead to insecurity, for instance, a lack of social protection, poor working conditions, a lack of autonomy over hours, poor pay and a general lack of job security (Vosko et al, 2009; Vosko, 2010; Campbell and Price, 2016). 'Precarious work' describes jobs that typically display a number of precarious employment characteristics, and therefore are not seen as 'good' jobs (Standing, 2011; Campbell and Price, 2016). For instance, roles with zero-hour contracts and with no pension, sickness or holiday pay above the statutory amount could be considered 'precarious work'. Such roles are prevalent in the adult social care and health care sectors. The term 'precarious workers' refers to individuals who engage in precarious work that has a significant impact on the security of their life (Anderson, 2010; Campbell and Price, 2016). For example, this could be older migrant female workers in the health and social care sectors on zero-hour contracts. The impact of engaging in this type of work could be an inability to purchase property, retire, have holidays or take sick leave. According to Standing (2011), the 'precariat' is a new class group that lacks security; the word originates from the Marxist notion of the working class, or the proletariat, spliced with the word precarity, to indicate a group attempting to climb up the class ladder (Campbell and Price, 2016). 'Precarity' refers to a more general notion of precarity, originating from employment conditions, but also seeping into housing, benefits and personal life (Anderson, 2010). This can also be linked to a sense of ontological precarity, whereby, according to Millar (2017), an individual's world view and understanding of reality is defined by experiences of precariousness. Therefore Millar (2017) suggests a relationship between Campbell and Price's (2016) notions of precarious work and precarious lifeworlds.

The underlying theories used here in relation to labour studies originate from two key authors: understandings of precarity as an existential condition can be linked back to the work of Butler (2004) and precarity as a class-based embodied habitus impacted by global economic conditions (like neoliberalism) originates from Bourdieu's (1998) work. Butler (2004) examines precarity as an inevitable human condition following the 11 September 2001 attacks on the World Trade Centre in New York. Her work attempts to counteract nationalistic discourses that justify increasing surveillance by claiming that it eradicates the vulnerability of human life. This is not to say that she argues for determinism and inaction in relation to the precarity of populations, but rather that feeling vulnerable leads to greater understanding and instils a sense of empathy for other people's less fortunate positions. Butler's (2004) argument is a political one, inasmuch as she argues that acts of violence are not individualistic but rather a product of particular discourses that shape policies and institutions. To examine why violent acts such as the Twin Tower attacks occurred is to take a step closer to understanding and readdressing the underlying inequalities (Butler, 2004). The neglectful rejection of vulnerability as a human condition enables the propagation of hierarchical understandings of who deserves to be protected and cared for and whose lives do not matter as much (Butler, 2004). In this sense, Butler argues, to understand precarity as a human condition protects the value of all human life. It aids the understanding of vulnerable groups, undermines violent backlashes and encourages investigations beyond individual action, which instead look towards broader political discourses and structures. Similarly, Bourdieu (1998) examines precarity within the context of wider political discourses, or 'doxa', such as globalisation and neoliberalism. His emphasis is on the processes by which European countries have been indoctrinated to accept neoliberalism as an inevitable development that rationally produces efficiencies and wealth, thus celebrating the economic and denigrating the social sphere. Casualisation, flexibilisation and the erosion of social protections in the welfare state have disenfranchised workers and eradicated their ability to resist the undermining of their job security (Bourdieu, 1998). Globalisation has added another level of competition for scarce jobs, so that those working in Europe now compete with workers on a global scale, and acts to further undermine working conditions, wages, security and workers' ability to resist (Bourdieu, 1998). Bourdieu sees these changes as structural violence, dished out by 'competent individuals', such as finance managers, company executives and economists, on individuals who are seen as 'incompetent' and thus deserving of suffering (Bourdieu, 1998). These theorists offer insight into the broader discourses of neoliberalism and globalisation and how they have produced precarity. They do not, however, relate this to older people.

Only a handful of researchers have applied the conceptualisation of precarity to older people (Grenier et al, 2017a, 2017b, 2020a; Lain et al, 2018). Lain (2018) developed Millar's (2017) conceptualisation of precarity as both the individual's relationship to the economic system and also their lived reality. Lain (2018) argues that to make full sense of the precarity of older people's lives, a number of domains need to be examined – specifically the labour market, the welfare state and the household. Lain's (2018) research, based on interviews with older people working in the hospitality and local government sectors, highlights that older people experience precarity in the welfare system because there are insufficient pensions. This is due to benefits such as Pension Credit being withdrawn, the raising of the pension age, 50 per cent reduction in unemployment and sickness benefits, and changes to private pensions. Due to changes to the welfare system, older people are also more likely to be forced into precarious employment. They may be at risk of redundancy and work in positions that are physically draining, stressful and require long hours, with little or no prospect of progression or finding alternative employment (Lain, 2018). Finally, in the last domain, Lain (2018) argues that older people experience precarity in the household, exacerbating precarity experienced in relation to employment and the welfare state. With the rise in divorce rates, complex family structures and single-parent families, along with the decline of home ownership in later life, increase in renting and outstanding mortgage debts, older people are more likely to feel the strain of the changes to the welfare state and employment institutions.

Similarly, Grenier et al (2020b) conceptualise precarity in relation to different spheres and, more generally, as a paradigm shift from welfare to active to precarious ageing. Between the 1950s and the 1980s, mandatory retirement meant that older people were welfare dependent once they reached retirement age. From the 1990s, neoliberalism and deregulation of employment protection and pension provision has led to an emphasis on extending working lives, participation in unpaid labour and the maintenance of independence (Grenier et al, 2020b). In contrast, since 2008, when the economic crisis hit, Grenier et al (2020b) argue that there has been an erosion of secure labour, increasing gaps emerging between generations and a weakening of rights to social protection in law. Furthermore, with an increase in the pension age, older people are more likely to have to find precarious employment or self-employment to bridge the gap between when they expected to retire and their new retirement age. Grenier et al (2020b) argue that the concept of precarity highlights the unwanted insecurity, hazards and risks caused by globalisation, neoliberalism and an undermining of social protections. They argue that the impact that precarity has on older people's lives includes getting stuck in a 'precarity trap', wherein older people are forced to remain or re-join the workforce; older people become more reliant on precarious workers as carers; families are undermined by the precarious labour market; and precarity has become institutionalised through the cutting of social and health care budgets (Grenier et al, 2020b).

Grenier et al (2020b) theorise that there are four indicators of precariousness: 'precarious working', 'precarious environments', 'precarious resources' and 'precarious deep old age'. Precarious working relates to the 'casualisation' of work and the shift to automation (Lain et al, 2020); 'precarious environments' relate to climate change and the injustices experienced by different populations (Settersten, 2020); 'precarious resources' refers to the deregulation of pension, health and social care provision (Macnicol, 2015); and 'precarious deep old age' reflects the increasing 'biomedicalisation' of older age, alongside the language and discourse of frailty and dementia (Grenier et al, 2017a, 2017b, 2020a). Instead of understanding notions of frailty as only applicable to people in later life, they argue, it should be conceptualised as something individuals experience throughout the lifecourse. Drawing on Butler's (2004) existential theorisation of precarity, Grenier et al (2020b) argue that frailty is an inevitable part of one's life and that this universalising understanding can destigmatise older people's experiences, by understanding frailty as a fluid experience rather than as something associated with the fourth age.

Conclusion

This chapter provides a theoretical underpinning for the ways in which ageing, capital, identities, vulnerabilities and precarity can be understood. Three main theoretical traditions have been used to illuminate the key concepts used in this book: those originating with Foucault's and Bourdieu's work, as well as feminist intersectional theory. Although these may seem incommensurable in their perspectives, these theoretical traditions have many overlapping analyses that are useful when it comes to understandings of how older people have become vulnerable and precarious in health and social care systems in the Global North. Instead of focussing on explanations that emphasise individual choices, biomedicine or lifestyle, theorists working in these traditions examine the impact of broad discursive and structural changes resulting from globalisation and neoliberalism. They critically examine how the state has shifted responsibility for health onto the individual, how the possession of different forms of capital advantage health outcomes, and how the layering of identities/inequalities has cumulative disadvantageous effects on ageing. Finally, they highlight how these developments amplify the precariousness of anyone experiencing frailty in a health and care system in the Global North. In the next chapter, the impact of neoliberalism and globalisation will be examined in relation to three different welfare state systems.

3

Globalisation, neoliberalism and welfare state models: a comparative analysis

Introduction

Chapter 2 reviewed a number of theoretical perspectives that provided critical lenses through which to frame the book's themes, including the impact of global and national developments on health and social care. This and the following chapters use theoretical perspectives to examine the key global challenges that face health and social care provision for older people. Globalisation and neoliberalism have significantly shaped and moulded welfare state systems in the Global North on a national level, including health and social care services. This is the case for all the various archetypal welfare state systems: the neoliberal/Anglo-Saxon model, the social-democratic/Scandinavian model, and the corporatist/continental European model (Esping-Andersen, 1990). The United Kingdom, Germany and Sweden are used to demonstrate how three archetypal welfare state systems have been affected by neoliberalisation, and the resulting privatisation of health and social care services. The shift in responsibility for health and social care from the state to the individual has re-established the very class inequalities which the welfare state was originally constructed to eradicate. This regressive reassertion of class inequalities impacts health and social policy, and exacerbates the precariousness of the most vulnerable. This is especially true for older women with low levels of capital. Neoliberalisation and privatisation have made health and social care systems vulnerable to any pressures exerted on them, for instance, austerity measures or a pandemic.

Globalisation and neoliberalism

Globalisation is a frequently used, yet complex and contested term (Hyde and Higgs, 2017). In this book, globalisation has not replaced national-level analysis; instead, globalisation and the nation-state are theorised as interacting and shaping each other (Hyde and Higgs, 2017). It is argued that the reason globalisation has grown in power and ubiquity is due to the lack of any viable social-democratic political alternatives to capitalism (Beck, 1999).

Thus, the rise of globalisation has been argued to be inextricably linked to the collapse of the Soviet Union and the rise of neoliberal free-market politics (Beck, 1999).

Although the changes associated with globalisation are generally accepted, there are questions over whether these are 'new' or if similar characteristics can be seen at other points in history, for example during colonialism (Bisley, 2007). Many of the so-called characteristics of globalisation are arguably continuations of existing patterns and practices, including, for example, the exportation of jobs to countries with the lowest labour costs and employment protections; the impact of technology on time and space so that goods and services can be fragmented and produced across the world; transnational corporations creating divisions between countries to gain more profit; and global elites choosing where to produce, invest, live and educate their children (Beck, 1999). Essentially, these characteristics, and globalisation more broadly, are replicated across time and space as periodic re-establishments of global exploitation along 'racial', national or ethnic divides.

This re-establishment or acceleration of global racial or transnational exploitation has impacted welfare state systems in the Global North, including health and social care services. It is the health and social care of those most vulnerable that has been affected the most by globalising trends, from the movement of labour to the impact of transnational organisations on structures of finance and undermining working conditions (Bisley, 2007). Beck (1999) would argue that the recent proliferation of power among the global elite and transnational companies is due to the absence of social-democratic political resistance. Communism, which once tempered capitalism as an economic structure that aimed to redistribute wealth, has disappeared (Beck, 1999). In its wake, neoliberal politics, the philosophical aims of which are diametrically opposed to socialism, have proliferated. Therefore, neoliberalism and globalisation are inextricably linked: they are both political as well as technological, economic and socio-cultural developments that have been in existence prior to late or post modernity (Beck, 1999). Globalisation and neoliberalism, as two entrenched yet resurgent systems of class and racial inequality, have come together in a context of highly sophisticated and complex advancements in finance and information technology. Within the context of post or late modernity, the impact of these political, economic and socio-cultural changes have occurred at a speed and breadth never seen before (Bauman, 1998). It is the rapid expansion of systems of inequality that is unique to the era of globalisation.

A key feature of these highly sophisticated and complex financial advancements is the outsourcing of previously publicly funded services, such as care homes, to private organisations, also known as 'financialization' (Horton, 2019). This trend in selling off state-owned assets began in the

UK with the incumbent government of Margaret Thatcher at the end of the 1970s. Thatcher's brand of neoliberalism began with the privatisation of the utility companies, like those in charge of the railways, gas, and telecom, then progressed into outsourcing many other previously publicly run services, such as rubbish collection (Mazzucato, 2021). From the 1980s to the 2010s, governments tendered to private companies, bundling up large and complex state functions, such as welfare, prisons and probation, as packages of contracts to be delivered by third parties (Mazzucato, 2021). As is discussed in Chapter 4, first health and then social care was opened up to a mixed-market economy and in various degrees outsourced to private companies. One of the most notable examples of this took place in 2013, when Staffordshire County Council transferred 3,850 of its 4,000 employees to private shareholding companies that had been contracted to deliver all services including social care for older people (Brown, 2015). Although most of the public are aware of these developments, there has been no transparent public debate about the pros and cons of this radical departure from publicly run services, arguably due to the lack of political resistance to privatising low-status social care services (Horton, 2019). This large-scale outsourcing of public services has been justified on the basis that it increases competition and improves efficiency. However, governments have been accused of using outsourcing as a mechanism to shift blame and accountability from the state to the private sector (Whitfield, 2006; Mazzucato, 2021). Then, when things go wrong, it is not the government that has to take responsibility (see Chapter 6 for discussion of the COVID-19 pandemic). Furthermore, the franchising functions of the state have been proven to be socially wasteful and administratively inefficient, as the state must absorb any costs resulting from privatising services (Whitfield, 2006; Mazzucato, 2021). For example, in health and social care, when older people's needs cannot be catered to by outsourced organisations in the community, they are left in expensive hospital beds and labelled 'bed-blockers'. The complexity of interconnections in the global financial system allows transnational companies to hide their exploitative practices, rendering accountability almost impossible to pursue. Tracking the reach of the impact of financial transactions (where people are investing in a pension fund for instance) involves uncovering multiple layers of connected financial enterprises.

The other main criticism of outsourcing centres on the type of services on which private companies choose to capitalise. If it were the case that private companies drove through improved service provision and/or invested large amounts of capital into risky ventures, then profits would be justified (Bowman et al, 2015). However, running health and social care services is a low-risk opportunity for the private sector: the market will never run out of customers and does not require the investment of large amounts of capital (Burns et al, 2016a). Moreover, privately run companies often ensure profits by reducing costs in wages and eroding working conditions, leading to a reduction – not improvement – in service provision (Toynbee and Walker, 2020). Finally, outsourcing does not necessarily lead to good practice and decision-making. Arguably a codependent and quite dysfunctional relationship develops, wherein taxpayers' money supports organisations driven by self-interested shareholders who want short-term profits and who open up key public services to unnecessary risks (Horton, 2019).

So why – if it does not achieve any of the stated government aims or desires (i.e., if it does not lead to better-quality services, use taxpayers' funds more effectively or lead to accountability when things go wrong) – has outsourcing of public services been so swiftly implemented and maintained by governments in the Global North? One argument is that these are ideological rather than pragmatic decisions, demonstrating a commitment to the re-establishment of elite class power. However, first, it is important to consider the source from which this resurgence of racialised class power emerged.

The origins of neoliberalism

According to Cahill and Konings (2017), neoliberalist sentiment originated during the interwar period, when capitalism was going through an economic depression. They state that, at the time, socialism was considered a serious potential threat to liberalism. Therefore, liberalism was seen to have failed capitalism and neoliberalism was an attempt to rejuvenate the political ideology. Neoliberalists augmented liberal philosophy by arguing that 'natural laws of the market' were no longer central to the thesis, replaced by the reduction of inefficient state bureaucracy. Nevertheless, although the word 'neoliberalism' denotes a return to laissez-faire liberalism, minimal state intervention, and a shift of power from the nation-state to financial and economic global markets, this characterisation is simplistic and inaccurate (Cahill and Konings, 2017). Mirowski (2013) argues that neoliberal elites enforce market rule via states. He calls this the 'double truth doctrine'; governments have been deregulating and privatising public-sector organisations, while new regulatory policies and practices have been introduced to ensure market domination. Thus, the neoliberal project can be summarised as a paradigmatic shift from laissez-faire liberalism to the domination of the free market as the most efficient form of human organisation (Mirowski and Plehwe, 2009). However, according to Harvey (2005), this shift was instigated with the rise of Thatcher in the UK, Ronald Reagan in the US and Deng Xiaoping in China, as before the election of these key political figures, neoliberalism was a minority ideological tradition. Instead, Harvey (2005, in Hardin, 2014) argues that neoliberalism is a political discourse that emerged in reaction to 'stagflation' in the 1960s, used to restore sufficient accumulation of profits for the 'upper classes' and to increase inequality.

Therefore, Harvey's (2005) approach proposes that the second wave of neoliberalism in the 1980s was politically driven to re-establish wealth among the ruling classes. In the UK, it was the election of Thatcher under a mandate to curb union power and reform the economy to prevent stagnation. In the US, it was the election of Reagan, who planned to radically deregulate industry and weaken labour legislation while empowering financial institutions to stimulate the economy (Steger and Roy, 2010). Deng reacted to the prosperity of other non-communist states, such as Hong Kong, Singapore and South Korea, and, instead of implementing protectionism against this competition, shifted to market-socialist policies (Harvey, 2005). Zamora and Behrent (2016) argue that this rise in neoliberalism coincided with the dissolution of communism and the death of the socialist ideals of redistribution of wealth, public ownership of state services and provision of state benefits. This critique of collectivism, particularly coming from a few elite actors (Reagan, Thatcher and Deng), raised the profile of neoliberalism. It also changed its meaning, from describing a general shift from social-democratic policy to individualistic policies supportive of markets and business, into a concept at the centre of a strategic political project (Cahill and Konings, 2017). However, to Harvey (2005), neoliberalism was not a new paradigm, but instead the reincarnation of class power relations, sold under the smokescreen of empowering rhetoric, such as, 'choice', 'freedom' and 'rights' (Hardin, 2014). Neoliberalism has undercut policies that seek to progressively redistribute wealth and power to the working classes (i.e. the welfare state), with the aim of re-establishing class power via market elites, and it enforces these new powers through regulation (Harvey, 2005).

As with 'globalisation', 'neoliberalism' as a term has multiple meanings, to the extent that some argue it has lost its analytical usefulness (Clarke, 2008). However, Ong (2006) uses a Foucauldian lens to argue that there are different incarnations of neoliberalism that have been operationalised in different countries, thus context-dependent analysis is needed to examine the ways in which neoliberal biopolitical techniques have been applied to populations (see Chapter 2 for a discussion of biopolitics). How neoliberalism is articulated is contingent on which neoliberal ideas have been applied and which have been made exceptions (Ong, 2006). The application of exceptions to neoliberal ideology can be seen in the development of archetypal welfare state structures in the next section. Using examples from the UK, Sweden and Germany, the classic welfare state models, and their political and historical influences, will be discussed. However, neoliberalism is not only used as a theoretical tool; empirical data exploring the neoliberalised health and social care system in the UK are examined in Chapter 5.

Welfare state models and their political underpinnings

While it is acknowledged that Esping-Andersen's (1990) work is ethno- and andro-centric (Leitner, 2003; Walker and Wong, 2004), and has been subsequently superseded by other models, the rationale for its use, is to track the development of the archetypes over time, using three exemplar countries in Europe and the impact that neoliberalism has had on their welfare state policies (particularly health and social care). According to Esping-Andersen's (1990) original model, there were three main types of welfare states: the neoliberal/Anglo-Saxon model, the social-democratic/Scandinavian model, and the corporatist/continental European model. These three types are underpinned by classic political-economic theory. The neoliberal/Anglo-Saxon model is based on Adam Smith's notion of the market being the vehicle through which equality is achieved via competitive practice (Smith, 1776). In reaction to this, an alternative political position developed, based on Marxism and more authoritarian forms of welfare state policy; this was the Continental/European model. The final model, the social-democratic, broadly argued that there was a need for citizens to be healthy and educated within a capitalist system and advocated using social resources to emancipate the working classes (Esping-Andersen, 1990).

The social-democratic model is a good example of class-mobilisation theory, as it was based on the premise that the aim of welfare states was to redistribute class power through the transfer of capital or resources to the working classes (Shalev, 1983). However, class-mobilisation theory has been criticised for neglecting the influence that corporations have on state decision-making (Schmitter and Lembruch, 1979). Additionally, the influence that right-wing politics has had in curtailing the left's power has also been ignored (Esping-Andersen, 1990). Furthermore, class-mobilisation theory does not fit with countries that have welfare state policies underpinned by religious denominations, which tend to take a corporatist/Continental model (Schmidt, 1982). Arguably, only the Swedish model can be seen as a good example of mobilising classes through a welfare state system, and this does not ring true for other countries (Esping-Andersen, 1990).

Thus, according to Esping-Andersen (1990) in the neoliberal/Anglo-Saxon welfare state model, the underlying premise is based on the notion that alleviating and decommodifying individuals' need to sell their labour in a market-based system should be avoided, as this could emancipate them from the capitalist system. Instead, for countries with a neoliberal political tradition, it is more attractive to make workers heavily dependent on the markets and make it difficult for them to mobilise, thereby allowing the inequalities that exist in the market to play out between workers in a 'divide and rule' scenario between the 'haves' and the 'have nots'. This model of welfare consolidates market power, as the welfare state only steps in when individuals need a safety net. In operation, this model is means-tested, modest, has strict eligibility criteria and aims to stigmatise its recipients. Significantly, the state welcomes the market into welfare provision, either by guaranteeing a minimum number of service users or by contracting private companies to provide welfare, paid for by the state. However, the market cannot adequately provide social mobility, as it only caters for those who are already socially mobile and who have the resources to navigate it.

Germany represents the archetypal corporatist/continental European welfare state model, based on insurance schemes provided by mixed markets (including the state) offering significant benefits in return. Esping-Andersen (1990) argues that due to the dependency on contributions, these schemes do not decommodify individuals in the system, as they first must earn eligibility through participation in the marketplace, which in turn is dependent on a series of rules and regulations. Therefore, unlike the neoliberal/Anglo-Saxon model, the corporatist/continental welfare state is not obsessed with marketisation. In contrast, importance is placed on maintaining differential status, and the system provides very limited social mobility. In this model, rights are not disputed; instead, they are universal, and markets are on the periphery of provision. Furthermore, corporatist/Continental models are shaped by various denominations of the church and are strongly supportive of the role of traditional gender roles in childrearing; they thus also provide a safety net for families that have not fulfilled their 'natural' roles.

Esping-Andersen's (1990) third type of welfare state is the social-democratic/Scandinavian model. This model comes closest to decommodifying citizens, in the sense that it offers benefits at a level that gives individuals a genuine choice as to whether to participate in the labour market or not, without loss of earnings, loss of tenure or risk of discrimination when returning. This ideal welfare state scenario offers equal benefit to all, irrespective of prior contributions. Countries that adopted this type of welfare state are the smallest in number and have been politically shaped by social-democratic ideals advocating equality between the working and middle classes, and between the state and markets. Provision is not at a safety net level but is instead at an equal standard of living to the middle-class citizen. In many welfare states, however, opting out of the employment market is disincentivised through strict eligibility criteria, delays in the payment of benefits and/or restrictions on the period of cover.

Esping-Andersen (1990) argues that the development, allegiances and future of welfare states do not depend on their level of spending but on whom the structure benefits or serves. Minimalist neoliberal/Anglo-Saxon models provide benefits to the working classes and the most vulnerable, and recipients of benefits are often stigmatised by the middle classes. However, in corporatist/Continental European and social-democratic/Scandinavian models, the middle classes are also recipients of benefits and thus have a stake in ensuring the welfare state is properly resourced. Next, I turn to the modern-day structures and challenges in the countries operating the closest to these three archetypal welfare state systems: the UK (the neoliberal/Anglo-Saxon model), Germany (the corporatist/Continental European model) and Sweden (the social-democratic/Scandinavian model).

The UK welfare state system: a neoliberal/Anglo-Saxon archetype

The UK welfare state system was shaped by William Beveridge (1942), who identified the five 'giants' that welfare services should address: want, disease, ignorance, squalor and idleness. These needs were translated into the following government departments: Social Security, the NHS, Education, Housing and Regeneration, and Employment and Leisure. After World War II, in a time of relative political and economic stability, there was a strong consensual commitment among politicians to maintaining full employment and providing publicly funded services (Glasby, 2017). However, the financial instability of the 1970s led to the election of Thatcher as Prime Minister in 1979, and later Tony Blair in 1997 with New Labour's 'third way' politics. Both leaders applied the neoliberal ideology to the welfare state, introducing and emphasising the value of markets in diversifying the delivery of public-sector services using private and third-sector organisations (Glasby, 2017).

The neoliberal assumptions that underpinned these types of reforms were that the markets would deliver more efficient and cost-effective services for the user and the taxpayer, that the quality of care would increase, and that they would allow the system to be more responsive (Davies, 2017). Yet, the evidence suggests that markets are more costly and are difficult to regulate. Furthermore, they do not assure quality control of service provision. The conceptualisation of health and social care users as customers is also problematic when health and social care providers have their budgets cut by the central government, as happened, for instance, under the Conservative and Liberal Democrat Coalition Government's 2010 austerity policies (Bambra, 2019). The other main argument used to justify the marketisation of health services is that private-sector care is more efficient. However, evidence suggests that private organisations 'cherry-pick' the simple patients/operations/service provision, with the complex and more resource-intensive cases left to the public sector to treat and manage (Miller, 2007). Another assumption is that GPs are the best-placed professionals to financially manage services, by expanding community care they can ensure patients' care needs don't escalate and reduce the use of hospitals, which would save money (Glasby, 2017). However, GPs are medical professionals, not commissioners, and therefore may not have the skills, ability or will to be financial managers and regulators of NHS budgets (Glasby, 2017). Finally, the assumption that cash-strapped local authorities can bring their residential care budgets under control, when 35 per cent of care home beds are run by five conglomerates making up to 19 per cent profits on low-risk service provision, is also a fallacy (Harrington et al, 2017; see Chapter 4). These policies are not based on efficiency, effectiveness or quality of services, but on ideology. Another key neoliberal discourse is that of 'choice'. This has also been central to neoliberal health policy since the 1990s.

Competition, 'choice' and consumerism

Although neoliberal ideology has been in existence since the interwar period, as mentioned earlier, it started to take hold in the UK in the late 1970s with the election of Thatcher in 1979. The context in which her election took place was dominated by economic instability and strikes in industries that were significantly affected by global oil price rises. This marked the end of an era of relative stability and security (Cahill and Konigs, 2017). Antony Cosland's 1975 statement encapsulated a shift to financial restraint with the phrase 'the party is over' (Glasby, 2017: 36). Therefore, the predominant cross-party agreement to invest in public services and protect the right to employment was replaced with a neoliberal critique of public-sector expenditure. The neoliberal argument was that investment in state-funded services interfered with the natural mechanisms of a market, reduced efficiency and reduced the profits that could be invested in private organisations (Cahill and Konigs, 2017). Henceforth, business principles were applied to health and social care with the aim of increasing efficiency, paving the way for privatisation (Glasby, 2017).

Although the changes brought in by the Conservative government did not include integrating private organisations in health and social care provision, they loosely followed the recommendations of the review of the NHS by Roy Griffiths (then managing director of Sainsbury's) (Glasby, 2017). The integration of management functions and leadership were combined with the implementation of an internal market in which health authorities and GP-funding bodies would commission services from a number of self-governing NHS trusts (Hunter, 2008). A 'Working for patients' White Paper (DH, 1989b) was followed by another (delayed) report written by Griffiths (1988), and the 'Caring for people' White Paper (DH, 1989a) introduced similar changes to social care, with local government taking responsibility for commissioning and purchasing health and social care services. Local authorities were increasingly purchasing social services from a mixed-market economy, particularly when changes to social security led to significant investments in private nursing and residential care (Glasby, 2017).

The rhetoric of 'choice' and 'empowerment' was heavily critiqued by social democrats, even at these early stages of reform (Le Grand, 2007), as the responsibility for ensuring efficiency was shifted from the national government to local authorities, along with the requirement that 85 per cent of the new budget had to be spent in non-public sectors (Glasby, 2017). Finally, 'The patient's charter' (DH, 1991) provided a set of benchmarking standards so that both the public and the government could hold the providers of health and social care services to account. These measures set the foundation for a radical cultural transformation in health and social care, from one run and organised by medical professionals to one structured by competitive service provision, where managers commissioned discrete services in a mixed-market economy (Lund, 2007). It was also during the New Labour era that eligibility criteria for commissioning social care services in local authorities tightened; the Care Quality Commission (CQC) found in its 2009 review that 70 per cent of councils provided social care services to only those individuals with 'substantial' needs (CQC, 2010).

This agenda of marketisation was accelerated under the 'third way' politics of New Labour and its slogan 'what counts is what works' (DH, 1997: 11). Blair's 'pick and mix' style of politics operationalised itself in health and social care by increasing funding while encouraging the development of internal markets through competition and decentralising health and social care budgets (Walsh et al, 2000). With significant increases in funding came a proliferation of measuring and targeting of performance, alongside the development of clinical and care guidelines in consultation with service user groups. Although performance management frameworks were centralised, budget responsibility was decentralised to localities and primary care trusts that now commissioned 75 per cent of the health budget. In addition, competition was introduced by rewarding the best-performing hospitals with autonomy (Glasby, 2017). Another level of marketisation was introduced with New Labour in the form of independent treatment centres (ITCs), private organisations offering discrete treatments, such as hip replacements, to enable the patient to choose from a range of providers and reduce waiting times (Miller, 2007). In reality, ITCs were run by previously employed NHS clinicians, who cherry-picked the most profitable, low-risk operations to maximise profit and in 2007 were reduced in number because they were not economically efficient (Hunter, 2008). During this time, there was also 'an emphasis on quality, safety and clinical engagement', encapsulated by the NHS 'next stage review' conducted by the leading clinician Lord Darzi (DH, 2008b), overshadowed by the 2010 general election (Glasby, 2017: 40). Social care reforms implemented similar notions of 'choice' with the personalisation agenda, whereby adults were given allowances from the government to commission their own care services and manage them (Glasby, 2017). Having developed from a disability rights movement to improve the empowerment of disabled people in the system (Hunter, 2008), the personalisation agenda was arguably appropriated by governments to shift responsibility for care from the state to the individual (Ferguson, 2007). Furthermore, older people and their families did not necessarily want or have the capacity, to organise and manage health and social care (Glasby, 2017).

With the increased investment and central targets, health care strode forward, reducing waiting times, modernising buildings and improving health outcomes for particular conditions (Glasby, 2017). Nevertheless, some debated whether these improvements were enough to justify the investment; others questioned the role of markets and competitions in these successes, and argued that the presence of competition and collaboration within health and social care organisational relationships creates systemic conflicts of interest (Le Grand, 2007; Hunter, 2008). In adult social care, the personalisation agenda was somewhat curtailed due to the constraints of the financial crisis in 2007 (Glasby, 2017).

When a coalition of Conservative and Liberal Democrats formed the government in 2010, some policies from New Labour were continued, while others were transformed (Hunter, 2008). The White Paper 'Liberating the NHS' laid out the Coalition government's plan to abolish primary care trusts and health authorities, and instead to transfer the £80 billion budget to GP commissioners (who are effectively self-employed contractors for the NHS) (Glasby, 2017). In relation to social care, although the personalisation agenda remained unchanged, the new government commenced a review of the legal framework underpinning adult health and social care, which paved the way for the Health and Social Care Act of 2012. David Cameron's flagship policy of the 'Big Society' had honourable and relatively ambitious aims in the context of austerity, whereby he wanted to bring communities together and create a sense of solidarity and citizenship (Macmillan and Rees, 2007). But this policy was widely critiqued as an ideological smoke screen behind which 'communities' or individuals would be expected to take further responsibility for their health and social care by 'choosing' to help themselves (Glasby, 2017). Nevertheless, while simultaneously introducing further marketisation and emphasising individual responsibility or healthism (Crawford, 1980), New Labour also emphasised the opposite of competition: collaborative working and integrated services. These contradictory aims have continued into subsequent Conservative governments' health policies.

As previously mentioned, the reason for the scepticism towards Cameron's 'Big Society' agenda and associated policies was the timing and context in which it was introduced (Glasby, 2017). The extent of cuts to public services following the 2007–8 economic crisis was the most drastic implemented by any government since the post-war era (Alcock, 2010) and in the history of the NHS. The budget reductions in the NHS were significant and were made together with a demand for £30 billion in efficiency savings, which they argued was necessary due to the growing demand and expenses of an increasingly ageing population (Yeates et al, 2011). This was flanked with similarly aggressive reductions in local government budgets and has arguably changed local government forever: financial targets and waiting times have trumped quality of care (Bunting, 2020; Glasby, 2019). The reality for workers and service users in the health and social care services is that these cuts have exponentially increased tension at a time when demand and need is ever-increasing. This is arguably why a number of scandals have been exposed, such as the revelations of hundreds of deaths caused by neglect at Stafford Hospital (run by Mid Staffordshire NHS Foundation Trust) (Hunter, 2008; Bunting, 2020).

The National Audit Office (2014, 2015) and the Association of Directors of Adult Services (2014) issued several warnings about the impact of the significant cuts to public spending on health and social services, raising concerns about how increasing numbers of adults with more complex care needs were to be served when funding had undergone real-term cuts of 12 per cent between 2010 and 2014. In the financial year 2018–19, the NHS sector closed with an underlying deficit of £5 billion (National Health Service Improvement, 2019), which raised serious questions about its long-term viability.

The Swedish welfare state: a social-democratic/Scandinavian archetype

According to Esping-Andersen (1990), Sweden had survived de-industrialisation and recession due to investment in public services, particularly education and health, and by encouraging employment for everyone, including women. However, he also predicted that this model would produce a female-based social service workforce as women represent both the supply and demand in social service provision. For example, women need childcare services in order to participate in employment, but women are also the employees in childcare services. The Swedish system depends on two parents working, but pensions are given even for part-time workers. As previously stated, the future of this welfare state model depends on support from the middle classes, which means the services must keep up with the demands of middle-class families and expectations of technological developments. With its dependence on high taxes and full employment to ensure standards of public health care remain high, the Swedish welfare state does have inherent vulnerabilities, including its dependence on public-sector employment and having working-age individuals who pay the taxes needed to support the welfare state.

Esping-Andersen (1990) was right, however, to be cautious in this prediction for Sweden's welfare state policy, as Mishra (1999) discusses in a piece comparing Sweden and Germany as ideal alternatives to the Anglo-Saxon welfare model. In 1990, Sweden went through an economic crisis, resulting in full employment and public-sector investment being replaced by austerity measures and unemployment continuing to rise until the 2000s. Globalisation, and in particular the free movement of money, started influencing Sweden's economy and financial decision-making, with high national debt having repercussions on a national and global scale. Financial deregulation had empowered businesses to demand a relaxation of wage protections and working conditions, and to use threats of moving capital to foreign markets as a bargaining tool. In 1994, for instance, the insurance company Skandia (one of Sweden's largest companies) threatened to relocate out of the country if the Social Democratic Party raised taxes.

Mishra (1999) argues that wage equity, which largely existed due to the coordination of powerful employment organisations and the consensual approach to working conditions, meant that the market could be responsive and ensure high levels of employment. Once this was gone, wage variability increased, though still not to the levels in Anglo-Saxon countries. At the time, there was also no evidence of irregular working contracts apart from the state encouraging women to engage in part-time contracts. However, by the end of the 1990s, Sweden's welfare model was shifting from egalitarianism and good working conditions to wage variability and flexible working. Similarly, taxation went from highly progressive to moderate levels, with tax spending shifting from investment in state welfare to reducing the deficit.

Due to the cuts to taxation and disinvestment in state welfare, Mishra (1999) states, benefits were considerably reduced in the 1990s; sickness, unemployment and parental leave benefits were cut by 10 per cent and delays in receiving benefits were introduced, along with higher charges for prescriptions and a reduction in housing benefits. A 'workfare' policy was adopted, which required those seeking unemployment benefits to take part in compulsory training and work experience. Due to increasing rates of unemployment, some areas of Sweden paid social assistance well below the recommended amount. Finally, a number of changes were also made to pensions, with the middle classes increasingly being moved to private pension schemes, and both employees and employers being required to make contributions for the first time.

Mishra (1999) argues that there were obvious impacts of globalisation on the Swedish welfare state even from the late 1990s, including the undermining of full employment and centralised wage negotiations, and the reduction of benefits. Further, the withdrawal of Swedish capital had been fundamental to the destruction of citizenship and Swedish egalitarianism. As Mishra (1999: 80) writes, '[b]y denationalising the economy and providing capital with an "exit" option, globalisation has strengthened capital's hand immeasurably against labour'. Moreover, he rightly predicted that Sweden was not immune to neoliberal globalisation and privatisation in the coming decades.

Since the Swedish economic crisis of the 1990s, Krekula et al (2017) observe that the welfare state discourse has shifted from the idea that all citizens are entitled to certain benefits to focus on individual responsibilities and neoliberal citizenship. Reforms have been made to the welfare state because of a concern about the viability of benefits. This includes reforms to pensions, which were restructured in 2001 due to the perceived financial burden of an older population combined with people entering the workforce at a later age. The former pension system had calculated payments on the highest years of income, although the new system had a minimum level of benefit, payments were calculated as an average across all years of work. The minimum limit for retirement age was also raised from 61.8 for women and 62.7 for men in 1998, to 64.6 and 64.4 respectively in 2015 (Swedish Pensions Agency, 2016). Due to the higher proportion of part-time employment contracts in women's careers, this had a differential gender effect, with women receiving a higher proportion of the basic guaranteed pension and lower pension payments based on overall average earnings (Ojemark, 2016).

After the economic crisis of the 1990s, employment protection also radically changed, moving from high levels of income protection and centralised wage negotiations to flexible working and the promotion of low-skilled employment in the private sector (Davidsson, 2018). In summary, Davidsson (2018) argues, rising unemployment was addressed by deregulating contracts and lowering their quality, instead of creating more high-productivity roles and continuing with progressive class structural reform. This increase in private-sector employment has led to lower rates of collective bargaining for wages; however, the last-in, first-out principle has remained, meaning that established Swedish workers are protected, whereas newcomers (particularly those in irregular contracts) are not.

The Swedish health and social care system

As part of a social-democratic model of the welfare state, Sweden is known for looking after its older population and providing women with employment rights. However, even Sweden's health and social care services have been increasingly marketised by outsourcing key services to large multinational conglomerates making lucrative profits (Anttonen and Karsio, 2017; Meagher and Szebehely, 2019). Like the UK, Sweden first launched universal access to health and social care after World War II. Pollitt and Bouckaert (2011) argue that states that have built hierarchised and well-developed budgeting and management systems now have significantly marketised public services. It was because services were managed so well, that markets were easily introduced, with the aim of improving efficiency and choice in health and social services. So, although the role of commissioning remained public, services were provided privately (Anttonen and Karsio, 2017). During this first wave of marketisation in the 1990s, Sweden outsourced its public services and shifted to a 'customer choice' model of service provision (Meagher and Szebehely, 2019). In this model, service users' needs are assessed, after which they can choose a service from a list of providers and get tax rebates once they have purchased the services they require (Erlandsson et al, 2013; Anttonen and Karsio, 2017). However, unlike in the UK, Swedish social care services were not forced to outsource a percentage of the services (Anttonen and Karsio, 2017). Nevertheless, like in the UK, marketisation and 'free choice' policies were criticised for three reasons: first, the system was costly and did not save the government money; second, private companies were accused of cherry-picking the most lucrative services, leaving complex and costly services to the public sector; and third, questions were raised as to whether all individuals, regardless of age, social class and educational level, can make equally informed choices (Anttonen and Karsio, 2017).

In the 1990s, nearly all older people's health and social care services in Sweden were publicly owned. However, as a result of policy changes since this time, around a quarter of home care services and residential care homes are now privately provided (Anttonen and Karsio, 2017). Arguably, this 'hollowing out' of the state, and the fragmentation and divestment of the public sector, led to greater complexity in governance structures, accountability and accessibility (Rhodes, 1988; Anttonen and Karsio, 2017). Since the 1990 reforms, fewer people in later life receive social and health care in their homes (Sundstrom and Tortosa, 1999; Anderson and Karlberg, 2000). Furthermore, staffing in residential care settings has been significantly reduced, with many working on hourly contracts and with low competency levels (Stolt et al, 2011). In 2011, Triton, the largest for-profit organisation, faced a media scandal for providing poor-quality care and having high death rates among their older residents; it was subsequently restructured, rebranded and divided into Vardaga and Ambea (Harrington et al, 2017). Nevertheless, the Swedish government was largely seen as competent at governing these new markets, and older people's health and social care services are still publicly funded (Anttonen and Karsio, 2017).

The power of a few multinational corporations in Swedish health and social care markets, however, is significant (Erlandsson et al, 2013; Meagher and Szebehely, 2019). Their political influence in health and social care provision has led to tax avoidance by multinational corporations and more people working in the private sector (Rhodes, 1988; Brennan et al, 2012; Anttonen and Karsio, 2017). Additionally, because the private companies increasingly own or have built the accommodation, the Swedish government has less control over quality of care, profit-making and the placement of residents (Harrington et al, 2017). Furthermore, as service users have increasingly come to identify themselves as 'customers', they have become less willing to pay high taxes for public services (Anttonen and Karsio, 2017). This changed relationship with health and social care services, from user to customer, undermines the principles of inclusivity and equality (Anttonen and Karsio, 2017). Furthermore, the relationship between tax-paying citizens and service providers is undermined: Why pay taxes to the state if public services are provided by profit-making organisations? As a customer, it makes more sense to go straight to the service provider, as this gives the customer more control and accountability over the services being provided. These attitudinal changes, which have already been seen in neoliberal/Anglo-Saxon welfare states such as the UK and the United States, will perhaps now also be seen in Nordic countries, where increasing levels of privatisation are continuing to erode the right to health and social care (Anttonen and Karsio, 2017).

The German welfare state: a corporatist/Continental European archetype

The German welfare state model is different from both the UK and Sweden. For instance, in 1990, German law prohibited low-paid precarious employment. However, according to Esping-Andersen (1990), due to the German state's Catholic roots, women, alongside social services, were assumed to be the main providers of social care. Historically, there had been a lack of support for women's employment, yet Germany did offer good benefits for those who participated in enough paid work to be eligible. Although unemployment rates did rise in the 1990s, after the reunification of East and West, Germany remained committed to paying good wages, employment protection and unemployment benefit. Mishra (1999) argues that although these policies were embedded in law, businesses were keen to make the market more flexible to the needs of private interests. At the time, however, there was a growing market for irregular employment contracts and this was seen to be the answer to rising unemployment. Previously consensual partnerships between businesses and unions became seen as problems restricting the market, as they made it difficult to dismiss staff. Employers argued that, in the wake of globalisation, they needed more control over employment practices, wages and human resource decision-making. As with Sweden, Germany's businesses also threatened to pull their capital out of the country unless their demands to have more control over employees were met. In this respect, they seemed to have taken on a more neoliberal/Anglo-Saxon model, with the expansion of globalised financial actors buying shares in German businesses and putting more pressure on chief executives to produce profits.

According to Mishra (1999), the changes to income distribution were not vast but were growing. The greatest development was the disparity between stock market profits and wages. At the same time, top tax rates and taxes for businesses were cut (to avoid the outflow of capital to places like Luxembourg). In terms of social benefits, at the time both employers and employees contributed 20 per cent of wages for pensions, health care, unemployment benefits and sickness benefits, but this was dependent on a mainly male workforce (as you had to be working to receive the benefits) and family members (women) were considered caregivers. However, with unemployment rising and the growing irregular contract employment market, many were no longer able to access benefits (Clasen and Gould, 1995 in Mishra, 1999: 83). Still, there remained a commitment to the care of older people, as demonstrated by the introduction of a new compulsory long-term care scheme in 1995. Mishra (1999) states that unlike the UK and other European countries, by 1999, Germany had not made any reductions in social welfare. Nonetheless, after an election in 1994, demands were made to reduce spending on the welfare state to meet criteria set by the European Monetary Fund, and, like Sweden, a number of cuts were made to sickness benefits, pensions and unemployment benefits in order to reduce the budget deficit. These European criteria set out by the Maastricht treaty kept welfare spending low.

Mishra predicted in 1999 that any changes to the German welfare state would be gradual and not drastic, as the system had more support from businesses and the right wing because benefits were linked to insurance contributions. Germany had a strong economy, which also helped. Nonetheless, predictions were made about the impact the increasing pressure of globalisation would have on the demand to relax workplace protections. This placed employment protection and labour costs at risk, and increased pressure on the state to reduce welfare payments, demonstrating that perhaps not even Germany could avoid financial globalisation (Mishra, 1999).

After reunification, high unemployment rates followed between 2003 and 2005, which led to the Hartz reforms, targeting employment protections, and the rapid expansion of irregular flexible contracts or 'midi-jobs' (Hokema, 2017). 'Midi-jobs' are low-paid, part-time contracts; employees have the option to not pay into the pension and social insurance scheme, with employers only paying a fixed amount of social insurance (Jacobi and Kluve, 2007). These reforms can be summed up as shifting risk from the employer to the employee (Eichhorst and Hassel, 2018). Hokema (2017) argues that they also disproportionately affected women and older people, who were more likely to take on more precarious types of employment due to their caring responsibilities. However, Germany has also tried to counter this trend with a number of policies. These policies have ensured that those (usually women) who take periods of unpaid leave to look after relatives in need of long-term care do not lose out on pension eligibility and are supported with public long-term care insurance. Carers who work more than 15 hours a week can also take ten days of paid leave a year for sudden crises, with long-term pay insurance covering 90 per cent of income, and still get contributions to health, pension and unemployment insurance. Further reforms improved benefits for unpaid carers by allowing unpaid leave for six months in companies with over 25 employees, and access to interest-free loans. Finally, unpaid carers could reduce their employment for two years to 15 hours a week. Although unpaid carers would have to be supported by another income earner to take advantage of these changes, they go some way to provide flexibility, which benefits carers.

Under the Hartz reforms, unemployment benefits were also no longer provided to recipients at a standard of living comparable to their previous earnings; instead, a flat rate of benefit was paid, while the state facilitated access to work as much as possible (Eichhorst and Hassel, 2018). Unemployed skilled workers were expected to retrain and enter the employment market as soon as possible, whereas previously they had been encouraged to retain their skills and wait for an appropriate job (Hassel and Schiller, 2010). Employment centres were reframed as 'job centres' and were given more sanctioning abilities and responsibilities, including the ability to offer increasingly precarious or 'flexible' employment opportunities (Eichhorst and Hassel, 2018).

In relation to pensions, Hokema (2017) states that the earnings-linked public pension insurance scheme was still relatively generous, enabling retired people to maintain the living standards of their working lives. At the same time, occupational and private pension schemes, which had previously been relatively rare, started to grow. However, since reunification, the German government has made gradual changes to increase state contribution rates to the public pension scheme, to ensure it is fit for purpose. As a result, a number of changes were made to extend older people's working lives, including raising and equalising retirement ages for men and women. This included removing the ability for unemployed people to retire early, which it generally discouraged. The disability pension age was also increased to 63, with the eligibility criteria narrowed down. Some of the reforms were subsequently repealed due to their unpopularity with the electorate. Nevertheless, in 2001 reforms introduced reductions in pension income, undermining the golden rule that pensions would maintain former living standards; the government suggested the shortfall could be made up through private pensions (Schulze and Jochem, 2006).

The German health and social care system

According to Moran (1999), the health system in Germany was founded on characteristically corporatist traditions, establishing an insurance system as early as the 1890s, whereby doctors, insurance companies, patients and the state were all interdependent. Furthermore, the system was established to placate proletarian workers looking to form trade unions, by making health insurance compulsory. It was not until the post-war period that disparities in insurance schemes (linked to employment) were eradicated, with the introduction of a unified social insurance scheme. Both employers and employees contributed to this universal scheme equally, however, insurance companies were numerous and fragmented. So, there was a sense of equity between the employee and employer, while engaging with a privately run system. However, the elite, which purchased private health insurance, was exempt from paying social insurance. Thus, there were still disparities in the provision of health services.

Since the 1950s, however, according to Moran (1999), there have been multiple reforms to the system, which can be grouped into the following: firstly, a growing centralisation of health care organisation; secondly, political involvement in the delivery of health care; and thirdly, a shift from health care being free at the point of contact to a system wherein patients contribute to the costs of their treatment. These reforms were driven by a shift from industrial to late-industrial capitalism and the reunification of East and West Germany. Both developments led to mass unemployment of the working classes and to increasing economic and health inequalities. What followed was a growing introduction of markets and state regulation, both key characteristics of neoliberal politics. The introduction of customer choice, competitive tendering and pressure to derive profits from 'efficiency savings' are all policies emerging from the Health Care Structure Act of 1993. Subsequent discussions have also touched upon the rationing of health care services through a two-tier insurance system, in which basic procedures are covered in tier one, and additional health procedures are covered in tier two. These debates are, however, controversial, especially with reference to excluding health conditions linked to lifestyles and identities.

From 1994, all older people (and the rest of the population) were insured for health and social care costs (Busse and Riesberg, 2004). The process is transparent: older people apply to Medical Review Boards that assess the length and the level of care needed; if the application is rejected, an appeals process is available (Busse and Riesberg, 2004). Nevertheless, the health insurance reforms of the 1990s did lead to the marketisation of the residential and home-based care sector, however, the dominance of charities providing residential care has largely continued (Bahle, 2003; Grohls et al, 2015). Due to the decentralised political and financial structure, the provision of end of life care has received criticism for being patchy or non-existent (Buser et al, 2008), as has involving older patients in end of life care discussions in hospitals (Jox et al, 2010). Nevertheless, by law, older people have the right to choose whether care is provided by family, domiciliary, residential or ambulatory carers. Most choose to be cared for at home by family members, and 90 per cent of these carers are women (Bahle, 2003). Therefore, although marketisation has been implemented, due to efficient systemic organisation and legal protections, older people are unlikely to slip through the net like they do in the UK and possibly Sweden. However, despite attempts to professionalise care, women in the family are still most likely to be those 'doing' care for older people in Germany.

Conclusion

This chapter discusses the convergence of three archetypal welfare state systems (and in particular health and social care systems) with very distinctive histories. This convergence is characterised by efficiency-motivated state interventions that have facilitated market competition and customer choice while leading to growing disparities in access. According to Esping-Andersen's (1990) typology, the development of the UK health and social care system is unsurprising, considering that the neoliberal/Anglo-Saxon model was always based on the market being the vehicle through which equality, via competitive practice, can be achieved (Smith, 1776). However, when examining Germany as an archetypal example of the Continental/European model, it is evident that its original Marxist principles have been replaced by market competition and growing disparities of health and social care provision based on occupational status. Nevertheless, efficient health insurance systems and legal protections ensure that older people, in the main, are not neglected. Most surprising, however, are the developments in Sweden's health and social care system that, although still free at the point of access like in the UK, sought to find efficiencies by introducing markets into the tendering of health and social care providers and by giving 'choice' to customers. These changes have proven to be costly and to increase health inequalities, resulting in fewer older people being provided care in the home and the erosion of employment protections in residential settings.

This chapter demonstrates the pervasive nature of neoliberal political ideology and the impact it has had on welfare states in the Global North. As discussed, even those welfare states renowned for their social–democratic or class redistribution have been restructured around the fallacies of neoliberal efficiency – the idea that markets drive up quality, and the notion of 'free choice'. The implementation of this political ideology has been accelerated by rapid globalisation. Multinational conglomerates have spotted a cash cow in health and social care, and have moved to exploit this low–risk, high–return market wherever possible, whether that be health insurance, care homes, medical technology or pharmaceuticals (among others). These developments, however, have been to the detriment of older people as recipients of these services and products, as, in reality, many have little choice or ability to make informed choices. These changes have also been damaging to the staff working in these sectors, who have seen their pay and working conditions eroded in the pursuit of profit margins for stakeholders.

4

Failing health and social care in the UK: austerity, neoliberal ideology and precarity

Introduction

Historically, the UK, Germany and Sweden have been understood as the archetypes of three contrasting welfare state models. The structural convergences of all three countries' welfare systems have been driven by efficiency-motivated state interventions, market competition and customer choice, leading to growing disparities in access. This chapter will discuss the impact of these changes in more detail on a national policy level. The discussion will focus on the UK, setting the context for examining the individual experiences of older people and health care staff in Chapter 5. The chapter starts with a discussion of contemporary health and social care policy, including austerity policies. Following this, austerity measures will be considered in terms of the impact they had on the Health and Social Care Act 2012 and the Care Act 2014. The subsequent sections examine the privatisation of health and social care, focusing on the failure of two of the biggest privately run care conglomerates: Southern Cross and Four Seasons. Then the neoliberalisation of the home care sector will be considered, followed by a discussion of adult social and health care workers' precarity. Finally, the chapter will discuss the 'dementia tax' proposed by Theresa May's Conservative government, Brexit, as well as some of the initial health and social care policies under Boris Johnson's prime ministership.

Austerity policies

The 2007–8 global economic crisis led to a financial market crash, lower income tax revenues and higher public debt (Jack, 2017 in Glasby, 2019). In the lead up to the 2010 election, the Conservative Party blamed the financial crisis on what it described as New Labour's 'irresponsible' economic and fiscal policies, which included investment in public services (Lee, 2011). Further, David Cameron argued that public–sector investment had eroded the 'natural' individual characteristics of duty and responsibility (Lee, 2011). This political rhetoric contributed to the Conservatives' success at the polls, although they did not get an overall majority in Parliament (Bochel and Powell, 2016). The Liberal Democrats successfully pitched themselves as a viable alternative to the two main parties, gaining 24 per cent of the vote with eye-catching headline economic policies, such as the abolition of tuition fees (Bochel and Powell, 2016). Therefore, with a hung parliament, the Conservatives and the Liberal Democrats had to form a coalition. The Coalition government was in power between 2010 and 2015, followed by the Conservatives from 2015. Both these governments implemented a range of 'austerity measures' (Glasby, 2019), which the Coalition government initially called a 'deficit reduction programme' (Bochel and Powell, 2016). These policies took precedence over all others (Bochel and Powell, 2016). The Coalition government justified these policies by claiming that the previous government had spent all the money and overcommitted funding to public services, and that this had put the country's economy at risk (Lee, 2015). This narrative provided a convenient intellectual basis for dramatic cuts to public spending and shifted the blame for the financial crash from global neoliberalism to New Labour policy. From 2010 to 2016, the UK population was officially at the receiving end of austerity policies that were justified by scapegoating Labour for a global failure of the economic market system (2016 marks the point at which Theresa May succeeded David Cameron as Prime Minister and austerity formally ended, although the policy change was not distinctive).

The Health and Social Care Act 2012

Given the Conservative's criticism of New Labour's spending on public services and its role in the 2008 economic crisis (Lee, 2011), the introduction of the Health and Social Care Act 2012 demonstrated the ideological (increasing marketisation) rather than material (reducing the deficit) aim of austerity policy. During their 2010 campaign, the Conservatives announced that there would be no top-down restructuring of the NHS. However, once in power, they proceeded with a costly restructuring process, alongside a real-term cut in funding (Jarman and Greer, 2015). Additionally, Timmins (2012) argues, these changes were introduced at a time when the NHS was performing better than it had ever done in terms of waiting times and public satisfaction. Thus, the Health and Social Care Act of 2012 did not result in savings, but cost more money (estimated at £3 billion in start-up costs and £4.5 billion in running costs per year [Paton, 2014]). Additionally, they were warned that these changes would create disruption, inefficiencies and low staff morale (Paton, 2014). According to Timmins (2012), the circumstances under which this legislation was introduced therefore suggest that this was a politically motivated project to impose neoliberal principles of free markets and deregulation, leading to cuts in health and social care budgets. Then-Health Minister Andrew Langsley's flagship policy, aiming to implement choice and competition while enabling the NHS to contract with 'any willing provider', was met with significant resistance in Parliament. He consequently had to water down his initial proposals substantially. Nevertheless, this neoliberal restructuring of health and social care represents the most radical departure in policy since 1974, when local authority functions were transferred to health boards. The overwhelming criticism and dislike of the bill led to a pause (which was nearly unprecedented) for reflection, consultation and amendment. Eventually, after 1,000 amendments, the bill passed the House of Commons. As it entered the House of Lords, 400 public health doctors wrote an open letter in *The Daily Telegraph*, stating that the bill:

> ushers in a significantly heightened degree of commercialisation and marketisation that will fragment patient care; aggravate risks to individual patient safety; erode medical ethics and trust within the health system; widen health inequalities; waste much money on attempts to regulate and manage competition; and undermine the ability of the health system to respond effectively and efficiently to communicable disease outbreaks and other public health emergencies. (McKee et al, 2011, cited in Timmins, 2012: 103)

This was somewhat of a prophecy because although it faced further significant challenges and obstacles from the Lords and health professional organisations, the bill received Royal Assent in March 2012. It is still considered one of the most controversial pieces of legislation since the poll tax (Timmins, 2012). These concerns will be discussed in subsequent chapters, specifically in relation to how fragmentation, marketisation and commercialisation have negatively impacted older people's care (see Chapter 5 in particular).

The Care Act 2014

The Care Act 2014 was a coalition policy with honourable aims. It was a significant piece of legislation that updated a myriad of individual policies and placed a holistic conceptualisation of an individual's wellbeing and decision-making at the centre of local authority social care commissioning (Glasby, 2019). Another key feature of this legislation was its move away from process-driven 'services' to outcome-based approaches to care (Clements, 2017; see Chapter 7 for further discussion). Many aspects of this act improved the rights of individuals with care needs, particularly in respect to enabling adults' (patients and carers) access to work, education and ability to maintain or start personal relationships with family or friends (Clements, 2017; Glasby, 2019). Additionally, it legislated integrative working practices between local authorities and the NHS, for example, a charging structure was introduced that aimed to prevent delays in discharging older people from hospital (Clements, 2017). Some adults benefited from the control given to them to purchase their own care and thus exercised agency (Glasby, 2019). The personalisation agenda promotes individuals' 'choice' and 'control'; however, people's choices are shaped by social and cultural capital (Bourdieu, 1984). Those people with higher levels of education and social support, benefit disproportionately from an information-led, agentic, health decision-making process (Harrison and McDonald, 2008). Therefore, these kinds of policies act to exacerbate, not equalise, health outcomes between social classes, which is the overwhelming thrust of neoliberal ideology (see Chapter 3). Nonetheless, although the act was generally positively received, its implementation was severely hampered by the impact of austerity measures on local authority budgets (Tope, 2020).

Impact of austerity and neoliberal reform on service provision

The Coalition government's austerity policies and neoliberal reforms affected all publicly funded services including welfare, education and health care (Beech and Lee, 2015). Although the health budget was technically ringfenced (unlike the social care budget), the lack of investment to keep up with demand meant significant real-time cuts (Glasby, 2019). The decade of cuts to public spending hit health and social care particularly hard (Marmot et al, 2020). Due to the cuts local councils had to make to their budgets, 24 per cent of commissioning bodies could not meet the demand for care in 2017. Between 2010–11 and 2019–20, there was a 29 per cent real-term cut in funding to local government income, which translated into a 4 per cent overall cut in spending on care, although this is still the highest level of care spending since 2012–13 (National Audit Office, 2021).

According to the CQC's (2017) 'State of care' report, the impact of the lack of funding has been the introduction of rationing and a general reduction in the quality of care. This has affected all areas of care, from primary and secondary care to community care settings (mental and physical health services) (Marmot et al, 2020). Waiting time targets were routinely missed for accident and emergency (A&E), as were referral targets for cancer and other conditions needing treatment. Alongside this, cuts in mental health services have led to patients having to travel further from their homes to access treatment. Satisfaction rates for GP services have also been decreasing. According to the CQC (2017), staff held services together regardless of these challenges, but there is a limit to their physical and emotional resources (discussed further in this chapter). The progress made by New Labour's investment in health and social care services, for example improving waiting times, is gradually slipping away. This was further amplified by the COVID-19 pandemic which led to the cancellation of planned treatments (Gardner and Fraser, 2021) and disruption of social care services (see Chapter 6 for further discussion of COVID-19).

Failure of residential adult social care organisations

As outlined in Chapter 3, the 'Caring for people' White Paper (DH, 1989a) insisted that 85 per cent of local authority budgets had to be spent in non-public sectors (Glasby, 2017). Thatcher wanted to expand her ideological commitment to the marketisation of the welfare system with this radical reform, privatising the social care sector and reducing public spending (Scourfield, 2011). Previously, 80 per cent of budgets were spent on public-sector residential homes (Barron and West, 2017). This reversal of funding sources marketised and commodified social care, while leaving the responsibility for purchasing, providing and regulating care to the public sector (Barron and West, 2017). Thus, local authorities are responsible for ensuring those who need social care are provided for and for paying for social care, but nearly all of the beds must be sourced from the independent sector, which consists of a mix of for-profit and not-for-profit beds (Burns et al, 2016a). In the 1990s and 2000s, the number of care homes was reduced, due to local authority fees, rising costs and increasing regulation. A few companies capitalised on new financing arrangements available and bought up large sections of the care home market (Scourfield, 2011). By 2015–16, five large commercialised organisations were running chains accounting for 35 per cent of the beds for adults in residential care (Harrington et al, 2017). When the care homes crisis hit the headlines, these organisations blamed the government, arguing that insufficient funding was available. This argument, which dominated media discussion, was in the interest of these powerful organisations, as they wanted more money to be pumped into a profit-making system (Burns et al, 2016a). The issue, however, is not only about a lack of funding in the social care system, but also a question of how the money is being spent. These big chain organisations are registered in tax havens in the Channel Islands and are based on similar financial models as those developed in the private equity sector, where shareholders invest funds in high-risk, high-return, financial projects (like start-up companies) or bail out failing organisations (Harrington et al, 2017). This type of model is therefore inappropriate when applied to low-risk sectors like adult social care; this should be a low-return sector (Horton, 2019), yet these conglomerates are making up to 19 per cent profits (Harrington et al, 2017). Further to this, the structures of these organisations are so complex that it is difficult to ensure accountability for the flow of public funds. Thus, sophisticated corporate structures mean that tax payments are often avoided (Harrington et al, 2017).

The consequences of increased privatisation on older people themselves were considered concerning at the time, particularly the lack of accountability for public funds, the narrowing of care home choices and reduced security, in the sense that if a provider collapsed, they would be homeless, as local authorities had no contingency plans (Hudson, 2014, 2019). For instance, Player and Pollock (2001: 252) stated 'care will continue to be predicated on publicly unaccountable private provision where shareholders take priority'. Following the collapse of Southern Cross, the government did introduce 'market oversight', a system to warn local authorities of the possible financial failure of care organisations (Horton, 2019). Nevertheless, this process of 'caretelization', wherein large corporations dominate the care home sector by buying up and merging smaller organisations, has meant that in some areas only one care home provider is in operation (Scourfield, 2011). Furthermore, even contacting someone at a care home is complicated when organisations have quickly and frequently merged or been bought by larger organisations (Scourfield, 2011). For example, is it the local, regional or national office that is accountable? The power imbalance between older residents and multi-billion-pound multinational organisations is vast (Scourfield, 2011). The ways in which 'caretelization' played out will now be demonstrated through a discussion of the collapse of Southern Cross, one of the biggest care home providers.

The failure of Southern Cross

The failure of Southern Cross can in some ways be compared to the collapse of the financial services sector in 2007–8, insomuch as there were calls for the government to step in and bail out private organisations with public funds. But how and why did it get to the point where a large multinational organisation went into bankruptcy and was pleading for the UK government to bail them out? In 2002, Southern Cross was relatively modest in size and capacity, comprising around 140 sites (Wearden, 2011). Over the following decade, they expanded by 1000 per cent, seemingly motivated by profits (through increasing commodification and asset-stripping) rather than a desire to provide more older, vulnerable residents with dignity and quality care in later life (Goodley, 2011; Peston, 2011; Horton, 2019). In 2004, Southern Cross was itself bought by a private equity company, Blackstone, which then bought Southern Cross' landlord, Nursing Home Properties (NHP), which was in considerable debt (Wearden, 2011). Blackstone's aim was to turn Southern Cross into the UK's leading elder care provider (Wearden, 2011). In 2006, when Blackstone decided to float Southern Cross on the stock market, while also selling NHP to Delta Commercial

Company (owned by the Qatar Investment Authority), which then sold NHP's debt to investors as bonds (Wright, 2011). In 2007, Blackstone sold its remaining shares in Southern Cross, making a 400 per cent return on its investment (GMB, 2011). That same year, three members of the Southern Cross management team left the organisation, including chief executive Bill Colvin, who made £36.6 million when he sold his shares in the organisation (Wearden, 2011). These substantial rewards were not, however, signs of a stable company managing its finances responsibly for the good of its vulnerable residents. Rather, the company had taken out risky bridging loans for which, subsequently, it could not manage repayments, leading to emergency talks with its banks (Scourfield, 2011). The company hit another hurdle in 2011, when the companies that had invested in NHP and owned the care home buildings increased their rents to the point Southern Cross could no longer make the repayments (Kotecha, 2019). At this point, the chief executive resigned, and the company made a plea to the government for a bailout, which was not successful (Scourfield, 2011). Perversely, it is this type of situation, where a care chain fails and thousands of older vulnerable residents are about to be left homeless, in which investors have the potential to make the most profit (Burns et al, 2016a). Such is the neoliberal system that has replaced the original outcome for the service – good quality care for older people – with the entirely opposing outcome of short-term profit (Horton, 2019). The impact of this shift in focus – from quality services to profit – was demonstrated in hundreds of complaints about the substandard quality of care in Southern Cross care homes, with undercover documentaries detailing neglect of residents, accounts of violence being used against older people, and the fraudulent keeping of medical records (Scourfield, 2011). The CQC, which regulates the sector, closed down a number of Southern Cross care homes, declaring such measures a last resort (Wachman, 2011). Southern Cross, however, is not the only example of a care home company with a complex organisational structure and a board making risky financial management decisions on behalf of its stakeholders. Southern Cross is a product of the system, which has been privatised and deregulated at the expense of older people's wellbeing. The Four Seasons is another famous example of a large multinational care home provider having financial problems and going into administration.

Four Seasons

Four Seasons is like Southern Cross in many ways, and their stories have many similarities. In 1999, Four Seasons was a small Scottish residential care company. At this time, the company was bought by Alchemy Capital, which went on to sell it to Allianz Capital Partners in 2004, which in turn sold it to Three Delta in 2006. By this point, the company had already accumulated considerable debt (Burnes et al, 2016a). In 2006, a consortium of banks (including from the UK), lent Three Delta, a company with Qatari investors, £1.5 billion to buy Four Seasons. However, in 2007, Three Delta could not keep up with the profit targets and was going to file for bankruptcy (Waples and Marlow, 2009, cited in Scourfield, 2011). Thus, the consortium lost £800 million, while the aforementioned companies that had bought and sold Four Seasons made significant profits (Waples and Marlow, 2009, cited in Scourfield, 2011). Four Seasons had accumulated £1.5 billion worth of debt, with interest payments of £100 million per year, which translates to £100 per week per bed (Burns et al, 2016a). In 2008, Four Seasons owned 400 homes and provided 20,000 beds to older people in the UK. However, it was also servicing debts of £1.5 billion (Burns et al, 2016a). Four Seasons was restructured, with investors taking control of the organisation and banks writing off debt (Burns et al, 2016a). Then in 2012, a European private equity firm called Terra Firma, run by English financier and investor Guy Hands, bought Four Seasons in a 'debt-fuelled £824m deal' (Pilmer, 2019). The care group, however, went on to have continuing financial problems. These culminated in 2017, when Terra Firma capitulated and passed over control of Four Seasons to HC Global, a US hedge fund and the company's largest investor (Wilson, 2017). HC Global invested an initial £40 million, which was increased to £70 million (Peart, 2018). It also froze interest rates to maintain the stability of service for its residents in the winter of 2018 while going through another restructure (Peart, 2018). Then in May 2018, Four Seasons and HC Global agreed on a rescue deal under which ownership would be transferred to a new company controlled by creditors (Peart, 2018). After continuing to struggle to pay its debts over the winter of 2018, Four Seasons went into administration in April 2019. By this time, the company housed 1,700 residents and employed 20,000 staff (Pilmer, 2019). The group's medical director stated that this was the last stage in the restructuring process and that the company would be sold by the end of 2019 (Pilmer, 2019). However, its latest announcement on 14 June 2021 states it's still 'in administration' (Elli Finance (UK) Plc and Elli Investments Limited, 2021).

The financial problems of Southern Cross and Four Seasons are not isolated. The three remaining biggest care home companies in the UK, HC-One, Barchester and Care UK, are also all up for sale and struggling to find buyers, citing Brexit-related difficulties in selling commercial property and a lack of local authority publicly funded residents (Pilmer, 2019). The fact that this is a sector-wide crisis lends more evidence to Scourfield's (2011) 'caretelization' thesis that opening up public services to private equity investment – whereby high-risk financial decisions driven by profit are made regarding vulnerable older people's lives, security and wellbeing – does not serve the commissioners, taxpayers or older people themselves, only private stakeholders. As discussed above, narratives that focus solely on a lack of public investment and call for the state to bail out these large private equity conglomerates fail to address how these conglomerates operate (Burns et al, 2016a).

The residential care home market is also cyclical and counterproductive: individuals invest in pension funds that buy shares in private equity companies that own care homes, yet these care homes also receive funding from local authorities to provide care for the relatives of these same individuals. The care home profits are paid to the shareholders, but when there is no longer any money left in the organisation and the investors are no longer making profits, the state is asked to bail out the care home organisation. As they are private organisations, there is no requirement for them to publish their financial information, making accountability to UK taxpayers impossible (Harrington et al, 2017). Evidence that the quality of care being provided by for-profit organisations is being undermined by them being owned by private equity companies can be found in CQC inspection ratings, which are lower for privately run organisations in comparison to non-profit residential care providers across all five of the CQCs fundamental standards: safety, effectiveness, respect, needs being met and leadership of the organisation (Barron and West, 2017). These results are reflected internationally in multiple review studies, which have found that for-profit care homes provide lower-quality care, are less efficient, cost more and are less egalitarian (Mercille, 2017). Mercille (2017) attributes the higher costs to stakeholder profits and the payment of large bonuses and salaries to senior management. Companies then try to make up for these by cutting costs in other areas, specifically by paying low salaries and feeding residents low-cost food. Additionally, nursing and dementia care homes receive lower ratings for quality of care, attributed to the difficulties in the recruitment and retention of suitably qualified staff (Barron and West, 2017).

Changes to the domiciliary ('home care') sector

Domiciliary care provision, like residential care, has also been privatised, but the shift from public to private provision happened during the 2000s, over a decade after the privatisation of adult care in residential settings (Rubery et al, 2013). In 1999, only 25 per cent of local authorities placed the majority of their home care contracts with independent providers; in 2008, 77 per cent of local authorities allocated over 60 per cent of their budgets to the independent sector (Hughes et al, 2009). This is because the driver for the privatisation of home care (best value) was different from that which drove the residential care sector (requirement that 85 per cent local authority homes must be for-profit). It was New Labour's 'Best Value' commissioning policy (DH, 1998) – which stated that no preference should be given to public in-house services over the independent sector, and that 'best value' should be assessed using a standardised procurement procedure – that drove the privatisation of the home care sector (Rubery et al, 2013). The marketisation of this sector has led to the implementation of zero-hour contracts, a reduction in time with service users, fragmented working hours and reduced quality of care (Atkinson and Crozier, 2020). Thus, the other group that pays the cost of the current for-profit dominated domiciliary sector and residential homes is the mostly female and disproportionately Black and minority ethnic staff (Horton, 2019).

Precarious adult social care workers

The marketisation or 'caretelization' (Scourfield, 2011) of the care home and domiciliary care market since the 1980s, alongside the more recent drastic cuts to public service funding under austerity policies, has also severely impacted another powerless and precarious group: adult social care workers. According to the Department for Health and Social Care report on the 'Adult social care workforce in England' (2018: 33), in 2016–17, 56 per cent of home care workers were on zero-hour contracts and home care workers had a median hourly pay of £7.50. Further, home care workers on zero-hour contracts had a staff turnover rate of 28 per cent, in comparison to 23 per cent of workers on fixed contracts (DHSC, 2018: 33). Some adult social care domestic workers have had their contracts transferred from public to private organisations and been promised the retention of their working conditions but have in fact been made to sign new zero-hour contracts (Hayes, 2017). Thus, they have gone from employees with rights to equal pay, guaranteed hours, holiday and sick pay, to becoming casual workers with few rights or entitlements (Hayes, 2017; Atkinson and Crozier, 2020). Social care workers in both residential and domestic sectors are therefore low-paid and low-skilled, and are not in general provided with paid training. These underlying problems contribute to the sector's difficulty recruiting and retaining professional staff (Atkinson and Lucas, 2013; Skills for Care, 2017; Thorlby et al, 2018). Social care organisations in the independent (private and not-for-profit) sector pay 12 per cent and 32 per cent less in hourly wages for a care worker and senior care worker respectively than their local authority counterparts (Skills for Care, 2017). It is also estimated that 25 per cent more care workers working for local authorities are qualified at National Vocational Qualifications level two or above than those working in the independent sector, and that under half of the adult social care workforce has relevant social care qualifications (Skills for Care, 2017). The lack of permanent contracts, pension contributions and sick pay makes a career in social domiciliary work in the private sector particularly unattractive. Even with pay rises via the introduction of the minimum wage in 2016,

30 per cent of workers in 2018 were paid in the lowest pay decile, whereas in 2016 this was only 10 per cent of workers (Bottery et al, 2019). If adult care workers' ability to competently carry out their roles is undermined by their own lack of security and value, this is undoubtedly going to impact the quality of care provided to groups such as older people. This is borne out in some of the data from a qualitative study that interviewed care home managers about their levels of staffing and resources, and the impact these had on the quality of care:

> 'Quality of care? There is no quality of care because you just can't give them what they need ... by the time you've done with it ... then you've got to go to the next one.' (Provider 3)

> 'I used to go home very satisfied that I'd done the best that I could. Now it's frustration ... the lack of staff. You're lucky if you have the time to do what you need to do without just having that little bit extra to be able to sit and have a minute talking to them ... it's not care.' (Provider 13) (Atkinson and Lucas, 2013: 303)

With fewer resources, managers have had to make impossible decisions about staffing and care practices. The adult social care service has shortages in nearly every role, but these shortages are in line with the health service more generally at eight per cent (Skills for Care, 2017). A lack of staff retention is also a problem and has a detrimental effect on the continuity of care; the turnover rate across health and social care rose from 23.1 per cent in 2012–13 to 30.7 per cent in 2017–18 (Bottery et al, 2019). These long-term trends are getting worse, with average vacancy rates in both health and social care growing by 18 per cent between 2016–17 and 2017–18 (Bottery et al, 2019). These problems are not just the result of austerity and neoliberal policies justifying cuts to health and social care funding or the result of an ageing population; adult social care workers and nurse numbers are also likely to be impacted by Brexit, which will put off immigrant workers coming to and staying in the UK (Dayan, 2017). The COVID-19 pandemic has also amplified these staffing problems, with many demoralised, taken-for-granted and over-worked (Age UK, 2020). This was particularly true of social care workers, who in the first wave, felt excluded from the recognition that health care workers were receiving and felt undervalued (House of Commons, 2020).

Precarious health care workers

When it comes to the treatment of NHS workers, frontline staff have had their wages frozen and paramedics, for example, have also had their working rights and conditions undermined. Paramedics are often taken for granted in the health and social care system: if no other services are available, they are often relied upon as health care professionals who will take up the slack in the system. With the pressures on community care services, patients being 'cared for in the community' are often not properly attended to. Appointments with GPs, district nurses, physiotherapists and other health care professionals are hard to obtain, thus older people tend to be neglected. Paramedics' roles have been adapted to address these inadequacies in the system: they are no longer ambulance drivers, but rather substitute clinicians who are expected to triage patients to see if there are any other alternatives to taking them to a hospital (Chilton, 2004; O'Meara, 2009). They are required to signpost, treat, refer and counsel patients (Dickenson, 2011; College of Paramedics, 2015). These tasks require skills that were not in their job description but which have now become part of their everyday roles, and for which they do not receive any additional pay. In fact, their working conditions have arguably become more precarious (McCann et al, 2013).

Junior doctors are another group that came under attack by the Coalition and Conservative governments under austerity, with Jeremy Hunt (Health Minister between 2012 and 2018) attempting to change their contracts under the mantra of a 'seven-days-a-week' NHS. The proposed changes would require junior doctors to work longer hours, and evenings and weekends would no longer be categorised as 'unsocial', meaning that they would no longer require higher pay rates. These changes would therefore lead to a real-term cut in pay (Godlee, 2016). Although doctors and health care staff already worked seven days a week, there were lower staff levels on weekends and, in particular, there was a shortage of senior clinicians. Yet, instead of investing more money to increase these levels of senior supervision, Hunt sought to address the evening and weekend shortages by changing junior doctors' contracts (Godlee, 2016). In the process, junior doctors and nurses were blamed for the supposed failings in their service, rather than the government that cut public funds (Godlee, 2016). In addition, nurses, consultants, occupational therapists, physiotherapists and all other health care professionals had had their pay frozen for the previous six years under austerity, with some having to rely on housing benefits for their rent.

In 2019, Theresa May's government announced a second consecutive year of pay rises for public-sector staff, following eight years in which the wages of doctors, nurses and other public-sector workers did not go up (HM Treasury, 2019). This was likely in response to demands by NHS England, which had issued a number of warnings during the preceding winters. A&E departments were failing to see patients within 24 hours, with many (particularly older people) waiting on trolleys for hours until they were admitted. To avoid 'bed blocking', patients (again particularly older people) were also sometimes being discharged into unsuitable care provision settings that compromised dignity (for instance, by placing patients in mixed-sex wards) (Fisher, 2018). May's government was expecting to go into an election before the end of the year and it likely wanted to avoid a repeat of the winter of 2018–19, which Hunt had publicly admitted 'probably was the worst ever' in the NHS at that time (Fisher, 2018). This was especially urgent given that May's social care policy had arguably led to the Conservative government's reduced majority in the 2017 election.

The 'dementia tax' and the 2017 election

In spring 2017, May called a snap election with the aim of consolidating the Conservative government's majority in Parliament. Conservatives believed the results of the election to be a forgone conclusion, as they could not imagine losing, or even losing any seats, to the Labour Party under Jeremy Corbyn, who was seen as an ineffectual and non-serious contender (Asthana and Elgot, 2017). However, the Conservatives did not gauge the public mood correctly. The announcement of their so-called 'dementia tax' garnered a huge backlash from the public and culminated in the party losing its majority and withdrawing the policy (Asthana and Elgot, 2017). The social care policy at the time stipulated that an applicant assessed by the local council as needing social care would be classed as self-funded if their assets were over £23,250; this included their home, but only if no-one over 60 years or any other dependent (e.g. a child under 16 years or an ex-partner who is a lone parent) was living there (Glasby, 2019; Carney and Nash, 2020). However, the so-called 'dementia tax' proposed that in case of those who were deemed to need social care in their own homes and had property worth over £100,000, their property would be sold after their death to recoup the cost of the care they received (Asthana and Elgot, 2017). By contrast, if an older person had cancer, for instance, that would be assessed as a 'health' rather than 'social' care need and would be likely to be financed by the NHS (Carney and Nash, 2020). This is where the phrase 'dementia tax' originated; older people suffering from dementia are generally categorised as needing 'social care', and therefore are means-tested and would need to potentially self-fund, whereas if they were classed as having a 'health care' need, they wouldn't need to do so. It also meant that the house would not be exempt if the older person received domiciliary care at home, as was the case formerly. The net effect of this proposed policy would have been that deceased older people's homes (previously exempt) would be sold to pay for the social care costs, and potentially only £100,000 of the house sale would be passed onto the family in inheritance (Asthana and Elgot, 2017). This could be seen as testing the public's attitudes towards neoliberalism in action, in relation to this subtle policy shift in responsibility for funding social care in one's own home from the state to the individual (Crawford, 1980). However, since

2017, the public and political agenda has been dominated by other events, such as the UK exiting from the European Union in December 2019 (with a transition period ending December 2020) and the COVID-19 pandemic from March 2020.

Brexit and Boris

Since 2016, there have been numerous leadership and parliamentary elections linked to Brexit and, despite the importance the UK public placed on the NHS, there was concern that health and social care policy would be overshadowed by Brexit (Wellings, 2017; Murray, 2019). However, there did seem to be some acknowledgement of the political importance of health and social care, even prior to the COVID-19 pandemic. For instance, in September 2019 and March 2020, budgets increased spending on capital investment, public health, education and training, but this was not enough to restore the NHS to the point where it could deliver on waiting-time targets (The King's Fund, 2020):

> In July 2018, the NHS was given a new five-year funding deal that will see some health spending rise by 3.4 per cent on average from 2019/20 to 2023/24 … In the September 2019 Spending Round, the government announced further increases to budgets for capital investment, public health and the education and training of the NHS workforce. Even with these increases, the total Department of Health and Social Care budget will rise by 2.9 per cent between 2019/20 and 2020/21, which is less than both the long-run average and the rises that NHS England's mandate services will see. (The King's Fund, 2020)

When the NHS is under strain in its day-to-day running, investment in ringfenced areas like public health are redirected (The King's Fund, 2020). Notwithstanding, Brexit will exacerbate staffing shortages, particularly in social care, as social care workers from the EU are not eligible for the new Health and Social Care Visa (Holmes, 2021). Brexit meant an end to reciprocal health care arrangements for British citizens living in the EU, replaced with fragmented and complicated substitute arrangements (Holmes, 2021); which makes assessing the impact of this change on the NHS and social care resources unclear. The UK is no longer regulated by the European Medicines Agency (EMA), instead all medicines are now regulated by the UK Medicines and Healthcare Products Regulatory Agency (MHRA), leading to possible increases in medicine costs, as companies will have to duplicate efforts to gain access to both EU and UK markets (Holmes, 2021). Finally, the new trading relationships, yet to be established, will have an impact on economic growth and subsequent public spending on health and social care (Holmes, 2021).

From 2017 (until Autumn 2021), social care policy was seen as too politically dangerous to be addressed by the UK government; many policy reforms have been anticipated but not realised, apparently due to Brexit (Albert, 2019). In November 2019, the government announced a £1.1 billion increase in core spending for local authorities in 2020–21. Supposedly this funding was for adult care services, but it was not ringfenced (Phillips, 2019). This was seen to be inadequate and a short-term fix (Butler and Saper, 2020). Then COVID-19 hit underfunded, understaffed and mainly privatised care and residential homes in March 2020, the effects of which were devastating (Butler and Saper, 2020). Even before COVID-19, due to austerity measures, life expectancy had stagnated since 2011, and in 2015 had it decreased for the first time since the 1890s (Dorling, 2014; Hiam et al, 2018). The challenges borne out in the fragmentation of the health and social care system proved even more deadly than austerity in the UK. A consideration of how and why the COVID-19 pandemic proved so devastating for the most vulnerable and precarious (older people as well as health and social care staff) will be discussed further in Chapter 6, after considering the impact of neoliberal/austerity policy on the experiences of older people and staff in the health and social care system in the UK in Chapter 5.

Conclusion

The health and social care system has been described as having been privatised by stealth. Since New Labour came into power in 1997, private organisations have been encouraged to be part of the NHS in the United Kingdom. With New Labour's 'third way', a mixed-market economy was implemented in health and social care. This political philosophy aimed to incorporate social democracy alongside notions of 'choice' within a marketplace. In this way, services in organisations were held to account through a competitive marketplace system. If providers (whether private, public or third sector) did not meet the targets set for them, their contracts could be tendered out to other organisations. This is particularly true of community services, where a myriad of different providers all vie for the opportunity to provide services in the community.

Private tendering also took place in secondary care, where private hospitals, such as those run by Spire Healthcare, could offer NHS patients procedures, such as hip replacements or plastic surgeries, if they could guarantee shorter waiting times. The key difference here is that although these procedures were financed by the state, profits were going to stakeholders rather than being reinvested back into the public purse. This practice enabled private-sector organisations to cherry-pick patients needing the most straightforward, uncomplicated and low-risk surgical procedures, as these are the most profitable. The public sector is then left with the most complex patients suffering from multiple comorbidities. Treating these patients is invariably more time-consuming, resource-intensive and requires the most expertise. This is also the case in social care, where between 2015 and 2016, five large care organisations accounted for 35 per cent of the beds for adults in residential care, making up to 19 per cent of profits (Harrington et al, 2017). It might be considered a strange market in which private organisations should wish to invest. However, the reason these conglomerates have chosen to invest their stakeholders' money in social care is because it is a very low-risk investment. There will always be a need for older people to be cared for, either in their own homes or in residential settings. The local authority must by law ensure they are cared for properly. For instance, if a private organisation fails to make profits for their stakeholders and folds, local government must step in and provide this care regardless. One of the most infamous cases of a private organisation going bust and pleading for a government bailout was that of Southern Cross.

Since the economic crisis, however, austerity policies and associated cuts to public funds have eroded and undermined the ability of the health and social care system to provide good quality services to the public, and particularly to vulnerable groups, such as some older people. This has been highlighted during the COVID-19 pandemic, when thousands of older people have lost their lives unnecessarily. Nevertheless, even before this tragedy, health and social care services were struggling. Waiting times for routine operations were at a record level, older people were being left waiting for admission on hospital trolleys and accessing GP appointments has become increasingly difficult. The case studies presented in Chapter 5 are situated in this pre-COVID-19 context. They demonstrate how the pre-COVID-19 changes to national health and social care policy discussed in this chapter affected the care of older people and health staff in a number of settings, including public health, emergency care and end of life care.

5

Public health, emergency settings and end of life care

Introduction

Previous chapters have outlined the theoretical and conceptual frameworks underpinning this book. Chapter 2 laid out the theoretical groundwork, examining how neoliberal discourse has shaped global and national health and social care policies. A shift in health responsibilities, driven by the rhetoric of choice, has paved the way for the marketisation of health and social care systems in most countries in the Global North. The dominant discourses of ageing – biomedical, social-gerontological and the idea of 'successful ageing' – were subsequently discussed. The chapter went on to review concepts of capital and field as developed by Bourdieu, making the point that higher levels of capital can protect against precariousness in the field of health and social care. Following this, I discussed feminist intersectional analysis, together with the importance of how different identities related to gender, social class and ethnicity can produce inequalities that compound along the years of a person's lifecourse. Finally, the shift in ageing paradigms from welfare to active ageing to precarious ageing was discussed (Grenier et al, 2020).

Chapter 3 applied social theory to analyse global perspectives on the crisis in health and social care, particularly examining neoliberalism and globalisation, and their effect on health and social care models in countries in the Global North. Key concepts of competition, choice and consumerism were central to these discussions. Chapter 4 analysed national perspectives on health and social care in the UK, discussing the impact of globalisation and neoliberalism on health and social care policy. It discussed austerity policy and the ensuing erosion of social protections in relation to employment and working rights of health and social care staff. Both these chapters demonstrated how global changes through globalisation and neoliberalism have impacted nations' welfare states, health and social care systems, leading to marketisation, fragmentation and complexity, particularly in the UK.

This chapter links the global and national perspectives discussed in the previous chapters to individual empirical data in three case studies. The first two case studies (located in public health and pre-emergency care) employ different methodologies, which are detailed in appendices 1 and 2. All names used in them are pseudonyms. The research team for the second case study is acknowledged in Appendix 2. Case Study 3 (end-of-life care), is discussed using previously published work. However, first, the sphere of public or preventative health is examined through a discussion of 'active ageing' frameworks, which encourage older people to participate in physical activity. This case study exemplifies the 'active ageing' paradigm, discussing data collected before the onset of austerity policy in the UK, when precarity became institutionalised through the cutting of social and health care budgets (see Grenier et al, 2020 in Chapter 2).

Case Study 1: Preventing decline – active ageing and public health

'Active ageing' is an umbrella term that encompasses a range of policy frameworks and gerontological approaches, which often carry unintended moral undertones. The various conceptualisations of active ageing include positive ageing, healthy ageing and successful ageing (Timonen, 2016). Originally conceived to resist negative ageing narratives which associated older people with inevitable decline, active ageing narratives attempted to reframe ageing from stereotypes of worthlessness and decrepitude into more positive representations (Calasanti, 2015). Subsequently, however, it has been argued that such approaches have been hijacked by neoliberal governments that have appropriated the broad understanding of being active in later life. For example, active ageing originated as a WHO policy framework encompassing the integration of older people into several spheres, including, for example, being active in political life and the community (WHO, 2002). However, these aspects are rarely emphasised in policy schemas at a national level, often reduced instead to attempts to get older people to be physically active. Additionally, these policies make several assumptions regarding notions of individual freedom which are bound together with neoliberal thought. For example, they assume that older people can and want to be physically active.

This section illustrates how a group of older people have understood public health information provided to them by medical practitioners and physical activity professionals in the form of verbal medical advice and leaflets promoting physical activity in later life. As will be discussed, their reflections express frustration with the lack of attention active ageing policy frameworks pay to physical and socio-economic barriers. This highlights that levels of capital (material, educational, physical) shape older people's access to resources and power to achieve what may be described as a 'healthy habitus'. Furthermore, through questioning why older people 'should' discipline themselves to be 'healthy', 'active' subjects and citizens, the participants demonstrate resistance to the active ageing framework. In the interviews, different types of resistance to the classed, gendered and able-bodied subject positions being represented in the health promotion materials is evident.

There is evidence that the advice of medical professionals can influence older people's engagement in physical activities (Jimenez–Beatty Navarro et al, 2007). Foucault's concept of biopolitics (1978, see Chapter 2), will be used in this section to understand how discourses of active ageing have constructed subject positions of successful or unsuccessful agers according to whether they are able to be physically active. The section also examines how public health information – and more specifically, physical activity advice and information – given by medical and physical activity professionals is understood socially and emotionally, as well as the ways in which older people give 'expert' information to others.

This section draws on research that examined the barriers and benefits to older people participating in physical activity. Here, focus groups, interviews and diary data are presented, which explore experiences of physical activity in later life (for further discussion, see Simmonds, 2011). These will be used to illustrate the unintended consequences of active ageing policies and associated public health material. What became evident from this data was the impact that levels of cultural, social and physical capital have on people's ability to maintain 'active' lifestyles in later life (for further discussion, see Katz and Calasanti, 2015). For instance, older people's access to 'healthy' or 'active' lifestyles, and their ability to age actively is dependent on their levels of money and resources throughout the lifecourse. Nevertheless, participants in the research recounted a range of experiences of medical practitioners giving them public health advice that did not acknowledge these socio–economic barriers. Furthermore, guidance was narrower than focussing on just physical activity levels – one prominent piece of healthy living advice addressed the participant's weight and not their physical activity per se. Victoria's case illustrates her reaction to the emphasis her GP put on her weight:

Bethany: 'Is the most prominent message about your weight [rather] than about keeping fit or...'

Victoria: 'Yes, nobody says about being fit.'

Bethany: '...or even... helping your wellbeing generally?'

Victoria: '...using up some sugar so that helps with the diabetes, so I suppose there is a bit of wellbeing in that, but I think it is more aimed at your weight most of the time, that's what anybody ever says...' (Interview)

Healthy living advice, including about weight, has been used to regulate not only individual's bodies but whole populations (Lupton, 1995; Nettleton and Bunton, 2005). Older people have been targeted with health promotion policies and a relationship between lifestyle and preventing unsuccessful ageing has been established (Hepworth, 1995). Wright and Harwood (2009) applied the concept of biopolitics to obesity discourses. For instance, Foucault (1978) argues that discourses are constructed by power relations, producing regimes of truth, which limit what is sayable and doable. Wright and Harwood (2009) state that obesity discourse can be applied to populations to encourage individuals to work on themselves in terms of what they eat and do, for the good of their health, and the health of the population as a whole. Further, Wright and Harwood (2009) argue that discourses of obesity, which are constructed using moral dichotomies of 'good' versus 'bad' and 'pride' versus 'guilt'/'shame', are often internalised and have resulted in emotional responses like self-loathing, which can have a negative rather than positive impact on wellbeing. These feelings of shame were described by Victoria, who recalled an experience of a medical practitioner giving her healthy living advice:

'… you feel guilty if you are not doing something. I never used to think about it years ago, but, it is only just because … I know I am overweight, so the whole time that is on your mind, you say "oh well if I did more maybe I would" … I did go to the doctor once because I was putting on weight and I couldn't see any reason for it and I was being really careful with what I ate … and this doctor said to me, "oh there weren't any fat people that came out of Belsen [concentration camp] you must be eating too much."' (Interview)

When asked how this made her feel, Victoria replied:

'[G]uilty. Guilty because I don't like exercise, guilty because I am not doing [it] and guilty even when I am doing it, because I don't seem to be getting the results … you are not losing weight, you are not enjoying it and … I feel like these people that you see running around the streets that look like they are in agony and I think why are they doing it if they are in such discomfort? Obviously, they are hopefully getting something out of it but who knows why they are doing it. I mean I must be getting something from it, or I wouldn't go [to the gym] and do it and be also trying to think what else can I do that might be okay. I don't know.' (Interview)

Victoria was working on her body by attending gyms and continuing to exercise, despite her lack of enjoyment and lack of weight loss. Victoria's narrative elucidates how discourses of obesity and successful ageing have positioned her as an unsuccessful, guilty subject (Wright and Harwood, 2009). Compared with Victoria, Elizabeth acknowledged affirmation of her low weight by a medical practitioner:

'My doctor more than the consultant … you see … there was a lot of approbation when I went back about my leg … [to] check up on the break ... I had a lot of ... "you have really done very well it has mended beautifully", but in the same voice they would say "but of course most of that is because you are very fit and you don't carry any excess weight". That's what they said, and that was said not once but sort of several times and you know you get little asides like "thank goodness she is very light, there is no extra weight" and that was underlined I would think.' (Interview)

When asked how this made her feel, she replied: 'Pleased and a bit vain and I mean it was amazing.'

Elizabeth embodies the moral discourse of self-responsibility, which includes presumptions of self-discipline, restraint and self-mastery (Markula, 2003). As Lupton argues: 'Experts play an important role in mediating between the authorities and individuals' (Lupton, 1995: 10), as they use the normalised 'truth' discourses of successful or positive ageing to create 'good' and 'bad' subject positions. In addition to emphasising the importance of low weight for older populations, some participants experienced medical practitioners giving them specific advice on physical activity itself. For example, Joanne was told by a medical practitioner that she should continue being physically active even though she needed a knee replacement:

> [There was] No keep fit [today] – saw the knee specialist. He confirmed I should continue to exercise – but says I need a knee replacement. (Diary)

This was also the advice received from a physical activity professional: 'Pilates leader says I should try and continue to keep the knee moving'.

The suggestion that older people should continue to participate in physical activity regardless of levels of physical capital fits the active ageing discourse and is critiqued by scholars like Wearing and Wearing (1990), who emphasise the impact power structures and unequal access to resources have on people's ability to be active. Some physical activity guidance at the time was prescriptive, yet, not tailored to older people's corporeality, such as, the advice offered by the Department of Health's 'At least five times a week' policy, since superseded by its 2011 and 2019 physical activity guidelines, which were specifically written for older people and more recently for older people with different activity levels (DH, 2004, 2011, 2019). Evidence of these prescriptions are seen in Victoria's diary entry:

> We went to Felt Leisure Centre. Exercise is apparently what we all need to do. At least 30 minutes a day! (Diary)

Burrows et al (2005) state that some understandings of health are pervasive cultural and political discourses. This is the case with active ageing discourses. For example, Victoria came across a British Heart Foundation magazine in the gym:

> '… when I was going to that gym [I] picked up a magazine from the Heart Foundation which was out there on a coffee table, because… a girl I know has had a couple of heart attacks [and] I thought that she might be interested because you can have it sent to you free of charge. So it was quite interesting actually. It was a magazine and it was monthly or bimonthly and there was all sorts of articles in it about exercise, and keeping the heart healthy, and there was some recipes in there as well, but I thought it was quite good.' (Interview)

Victoria seems to have assimilated the advice and guidance from the British Heart Foundation magazine here. Nonetheless, older people also demonstrated resistance to organisations' calls for conformity to health policies. Participants such as Margaret (aged 64) stated that medical practitioners had attempted to give them information regarding physical activity:

> 'Oh yes the physio is always giving me stuff.' (Interview)

When asked if she felt it was useful, Margaret replied:

> 'No. Especially these stupid leaflets with little diagrams on, you know this leg should be here and that arm, oh God.' (Interview)

For some people, these types of instrumental approaches to the body are unappealing and they find it hard to imagine the benefits of repeatedly completing exercise and health regimes, being unable to find a meaningful link to their lives (Bury, 1991). Two participants, Margaret and Hamish, were both educated beyond secondary school level, and demonstrated high levels of cultural capital. This helped them to challenge the dominant active ageing discourse. Indeed, Hamish stated that he selected the information that he required from the healthy living leaflets available in his doctor's surgery, choosing what material to consume and what to ignore. This demonstrates the effect education can have on people's confidence:

> 'Oh I have seen them in there but I have just put them away. I don't sort of take them home, I think "oh yeah" and put them down, and of course the main thing I am interested in I suppose is about health and nutrition and about how things work. I look at that and study it up and then take what I want from it.' (Interview)

Biopolitics, and the influence of active ageing discourses, can be useful to understand how moral binaries construct subject positions – such as 'good' versus 'bad' and 'guilt' versus 'pride' – that older people embody. Nonetheless, possessing high levels of cultural capital enables older people to choose what health information they take on board and what they ignore. For instance, some older people did not find the leaflets useful at all or selected the information they felt was of use to them and ignored the rest. This demonstrates the power of cultural capital on individuals' abilities to resist and make informed decisions about consuming health-related information. As will be discussed in the next section, the importance of cultural capital was evident also in interviews and focus groups where participants were asked to reflect on representations of active older people.

Responses to images of active older people

Images of older people in the media are unrepresentative of people in later life, often depicting later life as a time of decline and degeneration (Centre for Ageing Better, 2020). This issue is not just confined to the Global North, but is a global phenomenon (Zhang et al, 2006). Moreover, older women are often absent from mainstream media images/representation. Images that do feature older women are often digitally enhanced to make them look younger, reflecting the depreciating value of ageing women in society (Calasanti, 2007; Hurd Clarke, 2010). Social media discourse conforms to negative stereotypes, such as 'old hag', 'little old lady', 'old codger', 'grumpy old man', 'senile', 'weak' and 'frail' (Centre for Ageing Better, 2020: 21). Even the trend of employing older models reaffirms cultural stereotypes of youthfulness and sexual attractiveness (Twigg, 2013). The emergence of positive ageing images was an attempt by some gerontologists to construct an alternative discourse through which older people are understood (Holstein, 2011). However, Wray (2003, 2004) has highlighted that 'success' is culturally and temporally defined. Moreover, despite attempts to create new and positive healthy ageing constructs, these images ironically create an 'other' unsuccessful mode of ageing: a subject position in binary opposition to what is conceived of as successful ageing by the state. This 'other' is characterised by decline and degeneration, which further perpetuates ageist attitudes towards those who have, for whatever reason, reached the fourth age (Laslett, 1989, see Chapter 2). Further, successful or positive ageing images can be seen as an attempt to delay or deny the ageing experience (Pickard, 2009; Lamb, 2014, see Chapter 2). For June, these images of positive ageing represented something inconceivable:

Bethany: '[Do] you think that [the leaflet] [see Appendix 3] would encourage you to be more active than you already are?'

June: 'Well you know I can't walk don't you? You know I have torn the ligaments in my leg and therefore I can hardly walk at the moment. I used to walk miles but I can't now.' (Interview)

With the rise of postmodernity and consumerism, there had been a shift to more positive images embodying leisure activities (Gilleard and Higgs, 2011). Perhaps some of these are also feeding on popular notions of older people migrating to rural areas, where they live happy, healthy lives (Hanlon and Poulin, 2021; see Appendix 3). However, for Harry, the images in the leaflets had no relevance:

'I don't take much notice of these leaflets I am afraid. I am not active enough am I?' (Interview)

This reaction exemplifies the gap between positive ageing notions of happy, healthy third-agers being active and Harry's embodied reality at 90 years of age. Furthermore, Margaret stated that such images are of people who are 'too young':

'Too young-looking as well. She just puts me off: too smug. That could have been put onto just one sheet.' (Interview)

Additionally, Harriet, also from a middle-class background, also identified personally with other positive ageing images:

'Yes. I think the cycling one and leaflet ones would appeal to me the most.' (Interview)

When asked why, she replied:

'Well, I can just imagine how that feels to be doing exercises like that.' (Interview)

In addition, members of a focus group said they felt the pictures represented older people in the third rather than the fourth age:

Patsy: 'I think you have got the wrong age group, Bethany.'
Hannah: 'I think … there are two age groups: there is the 60 to the 70 age group and then the 70 or older age group. I think by the time you are 75 the majority of those activities are only available to very few people. It doesn't make you want to be more active because you know you are past it

> ... the pictures on the front, they are just dreams, dreams of what I would have liked to have been 10 years ago ... we all wish we could. It isn't the case that we wouldn't.'

Patsy: 'We have just gone full circle with these that we can't do these things.' (Focus Group)

The third age is a life stage where physical activity and active engagement in social networks take place; the fourth age is characterised by dependency and decline (Gilleard and Higgs, 2011; Higgs and Gilleard, 2014, 2015). However, as Hannah states, the young–old, active, healthy embodied realities are only available to a minority of people at the age of 75. For most older men and women in the third and fourth age, images like those presented in healthy living leaflets (see Appendix 3 for example), represent the types of economic, social and cultural capital (Bourdieu, 1984) only possessed by a minority of older people. For example, Heather, who was from a middle-class background and was a professional physical activity leader throughout her life, said:

> 'I think I do more than a lot of people my age. Well, I never put weight on so I have been lucky really. I don't think that is a very good picture of the posture; they could have done it better from a different angle. Actually, it is a combination of two different postures which is neither one nor the other, it is part of [name of postures]. Anyway, physical activity and high blood pressure. Well, I have high blood pressure, but it is being controlled and I don't have any problems.' (Interview)

Instead of feeling too old to identify with the images, Heather felt able to utilise her professional experience and knowledge to critically evaluate the postures depicted in the images. In comparison to Heather, Patsy and Hannah had less cultural capital, occupied more traditional roles within the family and, due to their economic position throughout their lives, were not able to accumulate these kinds of educational resources.

Importance of representations of ageing in public health information

The accounts of older people's experiences of public health information in this section, arguably typified the 'active ageing' paradigm, which Grenier et al (2020b) described as dominating ageing discourse from the 1990s when neoliberalism and deregulation of employment protection and pension provision led to an emphasis on extending working lives, participation in unpaid labour and the maintenance of independence. Although the various conceptualisations of active ageing frameworks were originally conceived to resist negative ageing, by reframing ageing broadly in relation to social, cultural and spiritual activity, such approaches have been hijacked by neoliberal governments that have implemented a narrow interpretation focusing on physical activity in a bid to cut costs for the NHS. Thus, public health and physical activity information can be understood as an attempt to regulate older people's bodies. Medical practitioners and physical activity professionals (the 'experts') play a key role in this process, by mediating between the state and the individual, and by working to minimise state spending on health and social care services. However, when positive ageing images in public health leaflets were shown to participants (for an example, see Appendix 3), especially to those who consider themselves to be in the fourth age, they were described as irrelevant. Instead of working as a 'nudge', the images worked to position the participants into the category of 'unsuccessful older person', as someone potentially dependent on the state and perceived to be a drain on resources. Health promotion discourse assumes that older people are or will be dependent on the health service: '[t]he debate reflects oversimplified stereotypes and fixed age categories leading to "worst case" scenarios of the economic burden' on health and social care (Thornton, 2002: 308). The images could potentially have a negative effect on the emotional well-being of older people. Some older people with access to cultural capital were able to resist this regulation by constructing their chosen identities as physical activity 'experts' themselves.

In March 2021, the UK government published a policy paper detailing a new public health system that had the laudable aims of addressing inequitable health outcomes highlighted by the COVID-19 pandemic, stating: '[w]e will empower individuals to take greater control of their physical and mental health, through giving people tailored and targeted information, tools and support to make healthier choices throughout their lives' (DHSC, 2021a: n.p.). However, there remains a strong economic argument underpinning this rhetoric, citing the importance of health to productivity and the economy, while it simultaneously quoted the cost of ill health and pressures on health and social care (DHSC, 2021a). This neoliberal emphasis on individual responsibility, the economy and targeting information to make better choices reiterates the types of discourse discussed earlier in this section, with the same pitfalls. To avoid at least some of these unintended consequences, future public health campaigns will need to carefully consult a diverse mix of people in later life and address the well-documented entrenched structural barriers. The representation of older people in public health information and the tone of campaigns will need to utilise previously published information on what works, and place at the centre 'older people' as experts, for it to be successful. The next case study also examines the role of information provided to older people in relation to health care choices, but this time in pre-emergency settings.

Case Study 2: older people falling and being attended to by paramedics

This section presents a case study based on two sets of semi-structured interviews, together with observational fieldwork notes from a project examining the experiences of older people who have fallen and been attended to by paramedics (see Clarke et al, 2014 for research protocol, and Appendix 2 for qualitative methodology and acknowledgements of the project members). The data in this study was collected a few years into the UK's decade of austerity policy and arguably reflects the beginnings of a 'precarity paradigm', when social and health care budget cuts started to have repercussions (Grenier et al, 2020b, see Chapter 2). The first part focuses on the experiences of the older people and the second part focuses on the experiences of the paramedics. This data originates from a project that assessed the feasibility of an intervention aimed to identify those at risk of low-impact fracture. However, here the data is drawn on in order to illustrate the vulnerability of older people in the pre-emergency care setting. This is particularly true when an older person has had a fall and lacks the cognitive capital to remember health care information (sometimes this also included their carers).

Bourdieu (1986) theorised different forms of capital that contributed to embodied power, such as economic power (see Chapter 2). In the same way that economic power influences people's access to resources, cognitive capital also mediates health care decision-making. Labour theory uses the concept of cognitive capital to conceptualise the knowledge individuals possess that gives them the ability to choose services or products in a marketplace (Camerer and Hogarth, 1999). Here, instead, cognitive capital is being used to encapsulate the power of individuals when faced with emergency situations and how this impacts older people's ability to process, understand and remember information given to them by health care professionals. As health and social care services are decided upon in a market-based system, the ability (cognitive capital) to understand and weigh health information, and then make a choice is fundamental to health outcomes.

This section also examines how paramedics make decisions in the context of marketised health and social care. Paramedics used clinical decision-making skills in assessing, treating and triaging patients to community care by contacting GPs, social workers, care staff and family members. With triaging in responsibility to signpost older people to other health and social care services, they found it difficult to negotiate the fragmented system. The practice of not taking patients to hospital acquired increased legitimacy in 2005, when a nationally endorsed strategy was agreed to, and guidance was subsequently issued to paramedics that explicitly encouraged them to explore alternatives to hospital admission. In 1999, 30 per cent of 999 callers were not transported to hospital (Department of Health Statistical Service, 1999); by 2018 this figure had risen to around 50 per cent (NIHR, 2018). However, this change in focus was not all negative, when according to ambulance trust data, only ten per cent actually needed admission to an A&E department (AACE, 2011). Therefore, the guidance outlined when to take a patient to hospital, when to signpost them to another health care service, as well as when to treat them at home (National Health Service Confederation, 2014). Subsequently, paramedics have adopted the signposting activities and are treating greater numbers of older people in their homes (Dickinson et al, 2011). In sum, the paramedic's role has developed from transportation to an independent health care practice (Chilton, 2004; Givati et al, 2018). They are expected to provide health promotion and prevention advice, as well as immediate care (College of Paramedics, 2015). Paramedics are working as autonomous decision-makers, treating clinical problems and referring patients to other health care services (O'Meara, 2009; College of Paramedics, 2015).

Precarity of older people in emergency care

In the interviews, older people were asked about their experiences of having a fall and being attended to by paramedics. They were also asked whether they had fallen previously or subsequently, and whether they remembered being asked questions about their risk of having a lower-limb fracture. All participants had been assessed by the paramedics who attended to them to possess the mental capacity to consent or had family members/ friends who gave consent on their behalf and were interviewed instead. Nevertheless, some participants had difficulty remembering the experience of having a fall. Older people who fell in Sweden (with suspected hip fractures), and were attended by paramedics also felt very confused and suffered from impaired memory (Aronsson et al, 2013). Older people had trouble remembering information related to the emergency incident and the research project. In all health and social care services, access to treatment and ongoing care is mediated through different levels of capital (for instance, cognitive, social and economic) that impact an individual's ability to negotiate a complex system. When an older person is unable to recall information provided by paramedics, it makes informed decision-making regarding ongoing care difficult. Even some family members and friends of the older people who had fallen experienced fluctuating cognitive capital in these emergency settings. Therefore, there seem to be specific effects of being in an emergency health situation that inhibit people's cognitive ability and amplify their precarity (for a discussion of precarity, see Butler, 2004; Grenier et al, 2017a, 2017b, 2020a).

For instance, the first interview question asked participants to describe their experiences of falling and being attended to by paramedics. Some patients who were deemed by paramedics to have the mental capacity to consent at the time struggled to remember their experience of falling. For example, Frank stated:

'I don't remember much about it because when I have fallen before I have been fully conscious but this time I didn't know anything about it. I just found myself on the floor … I don't know if it was that lady or not, but whoever rang up for the ambulance I asked her if she was going to give me the kiss of life. I said "that would be a pleasure" but then the ambulance came and they took me in and I don't remember whatever happened in there. I haven't got a clue. It completely went from my mind. I don't know whether or not it is a psychological thing that I blank it out or whatever it was but that was it, I don't remember a thing about it. All I remember is I woke up. When I came to I was in the back of the ambulance and the chap says to me "oh you are alright there is nothing wrong" and whatever questions they asked me I must have answered while I was in there but I haven't got any recollection of it.' (Interview)

Out of the 14 patients who fell, one-third struggled to recall the incident and the paramedics attending them. Some of the participants also found it difficult to remember other occasions when they accessed health services. For example, George found he 'was a bit muddled' when asked about visiting his GP:

'I'm not sure whether I went as a matter of … I think I just went and said "have you, did you know about this?" and she, I think I had to go in any case, I think there was something else, and I can't remember what it was now. I'm a bit muddled in my mind. I can't remember whether I did have another problem. I had an irregular heartbeat and I think she'd said come and see me about that and then we talked about this at the same time … I think there was another reason why I went, otherwise I wouldn't have bothered her.' (Interview)

This was George's first fall and Frank had had two falls. The age range of these interviewees was also quite wide, suggesting that this temporary lack of cognitive capital can happen to people at different ages and with different experiences of falling. Many interviewees had comorbidities that complicated their falling experience (such as Parkinson's disease, heart conditions, stroke and musculoskeletal diseases such as spondylitis or rheumatoid arthritis). Experiencing multiple morbidities in later life renders individuals particularly vulnerable, especially when they find themselves in situations with heightened stress, like emergencies. This is encapsulated in the following excerpt from Natalie's narrative:

Bethany: 'So if you just start by telling me about your recent slip, trip or fall and what happened and everything?'

Natalie: 'Well, then two nights after that I had a stroke. A very minor one, I should think, because I regained my speech and my legs after about an hour or so. And then I was taken to [name of hospital] by ambulance. I wasn't kept in overnight; I was in the TIA [Transient Ischaemic Attack or "mini-stroke"] ward and then a couple of weeks after that I had a diabetic hypo [ph]. But I was on medication, which made me feel very unwell and I wasn't eating very much and I think that was the reason. You know, I'd never had one before.' (Interview)

De-emphasising falling experiences could be linked to perceptions of risk in later life, which are centred on the threat falling poses to their sense of self and identity (Ballanger and Payne, 2002, see Chapter 2). Natalie's attention was on her stroke and diabetes; her fall was understood as only one of the side effects of medication and not eating enough. The primary concern for many older people were the life-threatening events related to other comorbidities, not falling per se. It seems that the context of participants' lives and the presence of other life-threatening conditions potentially depleted their cognitive capital. This made it more challenging to engage with health-related material regarding their care and to operationalise their 'patient choice' regarding treatment, which in turn further increased their precarity (Butler, 2004; Grenier et al, 2017a, 2017b, 2020a). These themes were also present in the paramedics' interviews.

Older people's choice and sense of being a burden

While observing the care given to those who had fallen, and during the interviews with paramedics, older people's sense of reluctance to admit they needed help also became apparent. The older people who had fallen were embarrassed and desperate to get off the floor, in some cases spent several hours in the same position. They had reached a point of crisis and, with no other option, they had called the ambulance. Once the paramedics arrived, the patients wanted them to pick them up and let them get on with their life as independently as possible.

'It's very difficult sometimes … we certainly notice a generational difference because they've only called us at the last minute because they've been on the floor for hours and can't get up or because of an injury they can't get up, otherwise they wouldn't call us. They don't want us because they don't want to go to hospital.' (Alastair, interview)

Some older people who fall feel that they are a burden on the paramedics' time and do not feel worthy enough to be attended to.

'Getting them out of pain and getting them comfortable and making them feel important, not a nuisance, because a lot of them think of themselves as a nuisance, so it's really just making them feel happier and more comfortable … quite often they're always sorry, they're always sorry and you say, "well, it doesn't matter" … "But I am sorry, I'm such a nuisance" … "No, you're not" … whatever you say they don't listen … they do feel a burden.' (Sharon, interview)

Similarly, patients can choose what care they accept and seven paramedics out of 14 highlighted that some patients do not want to be referred to other agencies, have their furniture rearranged or take up treatments that they cannot see any benefits from.

'I mean, it's obviously important for them not to fall again but you can only help people as much as they want to be helped. There are certain people that you say, "you should move these rugs, you should do this, you should do that", and they come back, "well, this is my house, don't tell me what to do."' (Kerry, interview)

One 87-year-old patient who had fallen was on prescribed drugs for osteoporosis and had an alarm. The GP knew about her frequent falls and she had been referred to a falls prevention service.

The paramedics spoke to the patient's GP and confirmed that a falls prevention team had been to see the patient and she had exercises to do, which the patient confirmed she was not doing because they were too painful and hurt her hip. (Fieldwork notes)

Seven paramedics expressed that there was a limit to what could be done to help older people who fall if they do not want to be helped. Some paramedics suggested that many older people resisted help due to a fear of being moved into a residential care home. Such fears indicate the interconnectedness of health and social care in the minds of older people. Older people in the study wanted to maintain their independence, for fear of being placed in residential care. These wishes expressed by participants in the study are linked to connotations of being 'burdens' (Calasanti, 2020a, see Chapter 2). This narrative presents ageing as a process of inevitable decline and dependency on the state (Simmonds, 2011).

Signposting in a fractured system

Most paramedics reported that they referred patients to other agencies, services or individuals where possible to ensure that they would be provided with the best possible care. These included social services, community health teams, occupational health workers, mental health teams, GPs, out-of-hours doctors, nursing or residential homes, home care workers, and assisted housing managers. They explained how keen they were to refer patients to alternative agencies, but how they felt limited in where they could refer to:

'A lot of the community teams out there are so hard to reach. The community nurses, they're just hard to get hold off. Everything needs to go through a GP surgery and then you don't know if your message gets passed on … We can't do referrals to Occupational Therapy, which we, I think is something that we should be able to do.' (Katy, interview)

Paramedics emphasised that they managed risk on a case-by-case basis. In order to access alternative pathways to an emergency hospital admission, paramedics had to be sure that agencies were sufficiently engaged to ensure the safety of the individual.

'There is a lot more out there, so if they [older person who has fallen] don't want to go in, or they don't need to go in, you just need that safety net there, in a way just to cover our own backs as well, just to make sure that the patient's alright and the GP's aware and they get a care plan in place.' (Polly, interview)

They also reported that there were considerable barriers to interagency working and communication. This suggests that the fragmentation of the health and social care system has also made the negotiation of older people's care by health care professionals more challenging. Paramedics stated that they would refer patients into alternative care pathways when they felt this was appropriate and possible. Moreover, the majority of paramedics said that they would encourage a patient to inform their GP that they had had a fall, but that they would only directly inform the patient's GP if there was an unexplained medical reason for their fall. Furthermore, paramedics found that many falls occur out-of-hours so GPs would not be available at that time, therefore they understood telling the GP about the fall to be a matter of patient choice. However, bearing in mind the lack of cognitive capital that older people might have in these emergency situations, it is questionable whether they would be able to make informed treatment decisions at a later date about whether to contact their GP or not. Furthermore, even when the research participant information booklets had been left, some participants had not remembered receiving them and couldn't locate them. This raises the question of whether even leaving health information for patients to read, process and understand makes a significant difference. Furthermore, paramedics reported that many frequent fallers' GPs knew of their situation, and the patients were already taking osteoporosis medication and had been referred to a falls prevention service. For example, the following is an excerpt from my fieldwork notes:

22/08/2013 – 6am–6pm
… an 87-year-old female patient with Parkinson's who had fallen and couldn't get off the floor. The paramedic helped the patient off the floor and [to] go to the toilet, as she was desperate having been on the floor for a couple of hours.

Paramedics asked the patient how she was, patient said that she is fine, but feels like a bother. The patient also stated that she doesn't know how she fell. Paramedics reassured the patient that she is not a bother at all. Carer said she fell because she just gets up in the night without the Zimmer frame, as it doesn't fit around the toilet. Carer stated that the patient should have her alarm round her neck at night as well as in the daytime. The carer was concerned that she had to visit someone else that morning; the patient could have been on the floor for hours.

Paramedic asked questions about the patient's walking (whilst completing the Patient Care Report) and then asked the patient if she would like to go to hospital. The patient would rather stay at home. Whilst the paramedics are asking the patient questions, the patient starts to feel wobbly and patient states that this does happen sometimes. Carer states that patient had fallen before but hasn't hurt herself. Patient has vascular Parkinson's but has mental capacity. Paramedics explain what can be done to help with falls, treatment and occupational health. The paramedic then contacts the patient's GP to arrange a referral to a falls prevention service and to ask for a medical review.

Dignity is high on the paramedics' agenda; they make sure the curtains are closed before they start dressing the patient. Patient states that she would rather be dead than to live like this, paramedics are sympathetic but do not respond with any shock.

The paramedics spoke to the patient's GP and confirmed that a falls prevention team had been to see the patient and she had exercises to do, which the patient confirmed she was not doing because they were too painful and hurt her hip. The falls prevention team were coming back in a couple of weeks to reassess her. The GP stated that she had seen the patient recently but would arrange a home visit that afternoon. The paramedics spent one and a half hours with the patient. (Fieldwork notes)

Thus, even if paramedics and health professionals identify an older person as vulnerable, older people themselves may not identify with that label. Positivist approaches that record and attempt to minimise risk have worked to disassociate health care professionals' understandings of falls from the social context (Ballanger and Payne, 2002). In contrast, older people's perceptions of risk in later life are centred on the threat falling poses to their sense of self and identity; for example, being labelled 'a faller' can be experienced as 'infantilising' (Ballanger and Payne, 2002). Therefore, biomedical narratives are controversial in often failing to consider the social context or subjective experience of later life. Further, they encourage the construction of binary categories, such as functional/dysfunctional and normal/abnormal, into which the corporeal status of older people are placed. Moreover, through this categorisation and labelling of ageing bodies with aged stereotypes, social and economic marginalisation is reproduced (Krekula et al, 2018).

Precarity and making choices with older people in stressful, fragmented systems

This section demonstrates the complexity of decision-making that paramedics face when trying to understand and navigate the wider interorganisational context of fragmented health and social care services. It also illustrates that older people who have fallen are in stressful situations and may have limited cognitive capital, which could compromise their ability to make informed choices in the moment or even afterwards when information is left behind, as there is evidence of them not remembering even being given the research projects' participant information booklets. It highlights how older people often feel like they are a burden not only on health care professionals but on society more generally (see Chapter 2). This case study illuminates how precarious older people often are in the pre-emergency system; successful health outcomes are often dependent on having power and resources (in different guises) to negotiate access to the care needed. Family and friends who can act as advocates for older people and help them to recover in their home environments act as powerful sources of social capital. If older people and their friends and family are educated, they can use this cultural capital to read about services available in their area, better understand the eligibility criteria and weigh their health choices. For instance, Harrison and McDonald (2008) found that people with higher levels of education and social support benefit disproportionately from an information-led, agentic, health decision-making process (see Chapter 4). Economic capital also helps here as, for example, it can be used to buy in-home care services not being provided by the state to support older people. Older people who have fallen are resistant to being labelled as 'fallers' for fear of what this change in social identity would mean (Ballanger and Payne, 2002), as such labelling often reproduces social and economic marginalisation for them (Krekula et al, 2018, see Chapter 2).

Finally, as this case study demonstrates, finding a good space and time to discuss care options is important, as the moment when an older person is being attended to by emergency services is clearly not the right time for either the older person or their family member(s). The stressful nature of experiencing a fall that requires paramedic attention results in temporary confusion, impaired memory and lack of understanding about the situation (Aronsson et al, 2013). Older people can lack cognitive capital when they have fallen and are attended to by paramedics, therefore being in emergency spaces can amplify their precarity (Butler 2004; Grenier et al, 2017a, 2017b, 2020b, see Chapter 2). Paramedics, as health care professionals, are working in increasingly fragmented and complex health and social care systems. Marketisation of the system has led to a myriad of different services provided by public, third-sector and private organisations, all with different inclusion criteria, contact details and referral routes. Paramedics' roles now include signposting precarious older people to these services, which is time-consuming and arguably risky. This indicates a possible lack of support structure for paramedics in making reasonable clinical decisions outside of the standard protocols.

Case Study 3: negotiating end of life and advocating for the dying

Older patients navigating health and social care services at the end of their lives faced similar but slightly different challenges to those in pre-emergency settings who were attended to by paramedics after having fallen. On top of the complexity, fragmentation, duplication and inefficiency involved in triaging older patients to community care services, there was the stigma and taboo surrounding death. It is also another key health care setting that depends on the presence of advocates, such as friends or family, to act on behalf of older people. Making end of life care decisions are not always a priority for hospital staff, as doctors' modus operandi is to save lives, not to help patients die (Walter, 2020). Thus, although end of life care has received more attention recently, and non-interventional options are considered, many doctors do not have the training or time to conduct sensitive end of life conversations in hospital settings, as it is often quicker and easier to treat patients (DH, 2008a). Discharging patients into hospice care or their own homes with end of life services is also time-consuming and reliant on third-sector provision, which can be patchy and inconsistent (Wye et al, 2014). It is a postcode lottery as to whether a patient is in the right geographical area to receive end of life care services. Moreover, advocates are needed to guide them through the complex and patchy services available for them to 'choose'. Those from higher socio-economic groups have 'deluxe dying' experience in a hospice (Douglas, 1992: 579). Much like the 'no-care zones' described by Estes and Wallace (2010) in the United States, older people with the least capital in areas with patchy or non-existent services are the most vulnerable and the least likely to receive appropriate end of life care. Furthermore, end of life care has received criticism for not being accessible to minority groups, such as minority ethnic groups (Coupland et al, 2011) and lesbian, gay, bisexual and transgender (LGBT) groups (Harding et al, 2012). This section draws on the author's previously published work evaluating end of life care services, drawing on interviews with clinicians about end of life care conversations they have had while discharging older people from hospital. This case study uses data collected in the UK's austerity years and thus could be said to also be rooted in the 'precarious ageing' paradigm, at a time when cuts to health and social care had been institutionalised (Grenier et al, 2020).

Discussing death

Redwood et al (2020) have found that conversations about end of life care often do not happen in hospital settings for several reasons. These include clinicians being reticent to have difficult conversations about death being near and the consequences this holds for treatment. As a consultant in an MAU [Medical Admissions Unit] interviewed for Redwood et al's (2020) study expressed, such conversations are especially difficult for members of the medical profession, as they are trained to intervene in order to save lives:

> As a profession as a whole, the default setting for medics is to do things and it is going to take a bit of time to work out actually not doing things is equally good. (Redwood et al 2020: p 215, interview)

There is a cultural barrier in the ethos of the medical profession in relation to death: medicine is designed to prevent, cure or manage single diseases or conditions (Walter, 2020). Notwithstanding the shift from medical paternalism to patient choice following the neoliberalisation of healthcare, having conversations about how someone would like to die within this highly pressured and complex environment is a challenge (Walter, 2020). This is especially the case when end of life care plans are coproduced with family members, who are sometimes more reticent to discuss their loved one's death than the older person themselves (Walter, 2020).

Clinicians such as a consultant in an ED (Emergency Department) in Redwood et al's (2020) study suggested that a better setting for end of life conversations would be a calm environment where older people, their families and GPs could have those conversations in advance of hospital admission and construct a living will or advance care plan:

> We think these [end of life and resuscitation conversations] should be happening on an outpatient basis with our colleagues for patients with chronic illness or with their general practitioners, ideally. (…) I think it would be better had they happened previously when the patient was well but had obvious multiple chronic conditions that meant that cardiopulmonary resuscitation was not going to be appropriate. (Redwood et al 2020: 216, interview)

Furthermore, Seymour et al (2004) highlight older people's concerns about advance care planning. This includes not wanting to be asked about how they would like to end their life, being worried about how their families would react to discussing their loved one's death, the link that advance care planning has with euthanasia and concerns about changing their minds. Thus, these conversations are very delicate and need to be had with people whom the older person trusts (Seymour et al, 2005). Clinician's empathised with older people about how dissatisfactory it would be to have end of life conversations with someone you have just met after being admitted to hospital. As one consultant in an MAU put it:

> There are clearly patients who should not be resuscitated, and it's a difficult discussion to have in the cold light of day, but it should be had and it doesn't. And then actually it's a very poor experience for people when it has to be done in here [MAU]. (Redwood et al, 2020: 216, interview)

Inadequate information: fragmented IT systems

Even when older people have discussed and agreed on advance care plans with their families and GPs, communication of these to other health care professionals is also challenging (Walter, 2020). Wye et al (2016: 103) found that even in areas with an end of life care register where advance care plans can be kept up-to-date, GPs, hospital staff and paramedics had problems accessing the system, either because it was 'cumbersome' or due to 'technical difficulties'. The increasing fragmentation and complexity of health care systems result in vital information about older people's end of life wishes not being accessible, especially in an emergency (Walter, 2020). Furthermore, as independent businesses, GPs are under no obligation to update these types of registers, so they must be incentivised to do so (Wye et al, 2012). Finally, there are concerns about the social consequences of adding someone's details to the end of life care register, as it indicates their proximity to death (Wye et al, 2012). This, some fear, can lead to a form of 'social death' whereby medical professionals start to treat the person with less care and attention (Sudnow, 1967).

Lack of time and resources for sensitivity

Other reasons that prohibit end of life conversations from taking place in hospital situations include staff shortages and the pressure on hospital staff to meet targets on waiting times. Clinicians interviewed by Redwood et al (2020) felt that they did not have time to sit and sensitively talk to older people. Instead, an MAU consultant said that it was quicker to treat them with interventions:

> The junior doctor who (…) sees the ninety year old coming in [via the ED], struggling to breathe with a nasty chest infection has only so much time, so the easiest thing to do is to start them on antibiotics, start the oxygen and then they get passed on to MAU where the junior doctor there says okay (…) Typically, it's quicker to do things and not have the talk, because everything has to happen quickly, you have got to get people out otherwise you hit the [waiting time] targets. (…) So, there are perverse incentives that sometimes stop us from doing the right thing. (Redwood et al, 2020: 216, interview)

The bureaucratic nature of health care systems could be viewed through the lens of the concept of McDonaldization (Ritzer, 2018). As Walter (2020: 28) writes, 'around the world, organization after organization, like McDonald's, is characterized by efficiency, calculability, predictability, control and an irrational rationality'. Although it is more rational to have end of life care conversations to discuss the wishes of the dying person, managers, accountants and politicians have created health care systems that prioritise bodies being treated in a time-efficient and controllable manner rather than as human beings (Walter, 2020). The characteristic failure of bureaucratic systems to put patients' care at the centre can also be seen in the inconsistency of end of life care services.

Patchy and inconsistent community end of life care services

The marketisation of end of life care in the community also dehumanises and hierarchises people who are dying. Younger people who are dying of cancer 'before their time' are often more readily provided for in the community through interventions by third-sector organisations (Walter, 2020). Older people who are dying, however, are often not prioritised by organisations providing end of life care services, as this is considered to be 'natural' and more difficult to predict (Kessler et al, 2005; Walter, 2020). For instance, Wye et al (2012, 2014) found evidence that Marie Curie interventions to improve end of life care worked for cancer patients who were on fast-tracked care funding. However, patients can only qualify for fast-tracked care if they are predicted to die within six to eight weeks. This funding system, therefore, neglects older people's needs and devalues their lives.

End of life care services do not even exist in some areas of the UK, where there are effectively 'no-care zones' (Estes and Wallace, 2010). A postcode lottery determines older people's access to services that meet their needs, as organisations that do offer such services may not cover their localities (Wye et al, 2014). Even where interventions like the ones delivered by Marie Curie (evaluated in Wye et al, 2012, 2014, 2016) are available, they are threatened by lack of 'stability of funding, re-organisations, policy changes, burn-out, resignations, [and] fewer staff' (Wye et al, 2014: 11).

Advocating for the dying

A key finding of evaluations of Marie Curie's interventions to improve end of life care was the importance of the 'keyworker' (Wye et al, 2012, 2014, 2016). Due to the complexity of funding, services, eligibility and locality, having an advocate for the dying person at one of the most vulnerable times of their lives is essential to experiencing a 'good death' (Wye et al, 2012, 2014, 2016). This person needs to have knowledge and understanding of the end of life care systems and should preferably be a palliative care specialist:

> Services 'worked' primarily for those with cancer with 'fast track' funding who were close to death. Factors contributing to success included services staffed with experienced palliative care professionals with dedicated (and sufficient) time for difficult conversations with family carers, patients and/or clinical colleagues about death and the practicalities of caring for the dying. Using their formal and informal knowledge of the local healthcare system, they accessed community resources to support homecare and delivered excellent services. (Wye et al, 2014: 1)

End of life postcode lottery

This case study is an example of how older people are treated as 'bare life' when they come to the end of their lives; they are devalued and dehumanised in an end of life care system in which they do not fit (Waring and Bishop,

2020). Like hospital discharge (see Chapter 6), end of life care is undignified and inhumane, reducing people to '"unknown" and "ineligible" subjects and, in turn, professionals become "not responsible" for their care' (Waring and Bishop, 2020: 171). In hospital settings, bureaucratic systems, designed to enhance the efficiency with which older bodies are managed, disincentivise rational discussions about the suitability or desirability of interventions and mutual care planning (see Chapter 6). This McDonaldization (Ritzer, 2018) of older people's care is inhumane and neglectful. Even with the introduction of end of life care registers, where older people's prior wishes and desires can be documented, the fragmentation of health care organisations makes access to this vital information almost impossible. Clinicians understand the callous and inappropriate nature of older people's end of life treatment in hospital, but they work in health care organisations that are understaffed and have been underfunded for over a decade due to austerity policies (see Chapters 4 and 6). More recent increases in funding have not been adequate for these organisations to keep up with demand as well as technological and demographic change (Darzi, 2018).

The same can be said for the social care system; its privatisation, marketisation and commodification has resulted in threadbare end of life care services. In relation to end of life care, 'no-care zones' (Estes and Wallace, 2010) also exist in the UK, and this vital care is left to third-sector organisations with unstable funding. Where end of life care services are available, they are complex and difficult to navigate without a dedicated palliative care specialist to advocate for the older person (Wye et al, 2012, 2014). Criteria for accessing funding for services can also create hierarchies of need, where older people are placed at the bottom. Older people who are not diagnosed with a terminal illness (like cancer) often have a dying trajectory that lasts years (Walter, 2020) and, therefore, they do not qualify for end of life care (Wye et al, 2012). Furthermore, the intersectionality of ethnicity, sexuality and class add layers of exclusion to receiving end of life care (Douglas, 1992; Coupleland et al, 2011; Harding et al, 2012). Normalising death in later life as 'natural' and expected (Howarth, 2007) further legitimises the neglect and inhumane treatment of older people at the end of their lives. Arguably, this can be seen as part of the Global North's ageist culture, in which older people's lives are worth less (see Chapter 6).

Conclusion

What draws the first two case studies together is the importance of the presence or absence of different types of capital and the impact that this has on older people's ability to use health information to negotiate an increasingly complex health and social care system. Organisations that propagate public health information to get older people physically active dismiss the impact that social, physical, cultural and economic capital has on their ability to be active, especially when trying to replicate some of the aspirational activities represented (e.g. sailing, yoga). This is also gendered; with the feminisation of ageing (due to the difference in life expectancy, the percentage of older women outweighs the number of older men) and its influences on pension income and morbidity (Arber and Ginn, 1994), women are more likely to be the targets of these types of preventative public health campaigns. Demonstrated in the data are the often-counterproductive subject positions constructed; older people feel guilty and like they are failing at being an ideal older person if they cannot emulate successful ageing representations. Most importantly, this data illustrates the impact of intersecting inequalities on people's ability to be physically active in later life. Therefore, although the data presented here was captured before the COVID-19 pandemic, it has salient findings. Public health initiatives implemented because of COVID-19 must acknowledge these structural factors when trying to increase physical activity and reduce obesity (Marmot et al, 2020, see Chapter 6). Public health campaigns will need to represent the diversity of identities in later life, utilise previously published information on what works and place at the centre 'older people' as experts for it to be successful.

Older people are also given information (either verbally or on paper) when attended by paramedics after a fall. Paramedics are encouraged to signpost older people to alternative services in the community (public, third sector or private); older people are asked to visit their GPs and are canvassed on their choice of service. However, as demonstrated by the data, emergency situations are extremely stressful for older people and their family or friends; they often do not process information well or remember the events afterwards. Arguably, people sometimes lack cognitive capital in these particular times and spaces. This makes informed decision-making about these 'choices' very difficult. A lack of cognitive capital can be exacerbated by a lack of physical capital (such as having multiple conditions) and a lack of social capital (such as not having family or friends who can support the older person at home). Furthermore, although their levels of cultural capital have increased, paramedics find navigating the health and social care system challenging; interagency communication and continuity of care have been made difficult by increased marketisation and fragmentation, and there are no longer clear care pathways to follow.

Further, although hospitals are not always beneficial environments for older people to be in, being cared for in the community is also not always a good solution for older people who do not have the social and economic capital to recover from falls. Nevertheless, in a bid to save health and social care funds, policies like 'care in the community' and 'ageing in place' have been promoted to support older people through community networks and thus prevent an escalation of care needs (Settersten, 2020). However, austerity measures have translated into substantial cuts in community and social care, exposing older people to greater precarity in health and social care systems, with increasing levels of unmet need (Phillipson, 2020a; National Audit Office, 2021). This is especially the case among the most vulnerable, the 'oldest old' people or fourth-agers, whose mortality rates increased between 2015 and 2019, resulting in life expectancy stagnating for the first time in the post-war era and, in case of older women, actually decreasing (Green et al, 2017; Hiam et al, 2018; Raleigh, 2019). The COVID-19 Marmot Review (Marmot et al, 2020) examined the association of austerity and life expectancy over the ten years starting from 2010 when austerity policies dominated, and it reported that in most areas of deprivation north of London, life expectancy decreased. Further, Crawford et al (2020) suggest that the impact of cuts to social care funding has disproportionately affected older people from deprived backgrounds, with a third more people aged over 65 being admitted to A&E between 2009−10 and 2017−18, with 25 per cent of this rise being attributed to cuts.

Waring and Bishop (2020) use Foucault's concept of biopower (1978) to argue that state institutions produce deserving or underserving older citizens. This production of older people as citizens who are undeserving of adequate health, social and end of life care can be seen in Case Study 3 discussed in this chapter. Once older people are labelled as 'frail', they are marginalised and treated with pity rather than with an understanding of the universalism of vulnerability (Grenier et al, 2017a). Arguably, throughout the lifecourse, everyone experiences levels of precarity and risk (Grenier et al, 2017a). As Butler (2004) theorises, precarity is part of the human condition. This case study also illuminates what happens to the care of older people when social-cultural processes of discrimination towards 'the frail' (Grenier et al, 2017a) collide with austerity measures and rationing of social welfare (Phillipson, 2015). Bourdieu's (1998) theorisation of precarity and the impact of neoliberalism and globalisation is pertinent here too; the UK has been indoctrinated into celebrating the 'economic' and denigrating the 'social' sphere. The changes made to the health and social care sector, and the impact these have had on older people, could be seen as inflicting structural violence, dished out by 'competent individuals' (such as finance managers, company executives and economists) on individuals who are seen as 'incompetent' and thus deserving of suffering (Bourdieu, 1998). This is notwithstanding the intersectionality of inequalities such as social class (access to economic, social and cultural capital), ethnicity (linked to social class and racial discrimination) and gender (women being more likely to reach older age and experience 'frailty') that impact on older people's ability to exercise agency, either individually or by proxy, in health and social care settings (see Chapters 2 and 6).

Finally, although the data presented here was captured prior to the COVID-19 pandemic, it has important inferences. During the COVID-19 pandemic, paramedics, as 'key workers' have been at the highest risk of contagion, yet, the pressure of need among (particularly older) patients has been growing (WBG, 2020). Therefore, the already stressful context in which decision-making with older people takes place would have been amplified many times over. This chapter also discussed themes in relation to end of life care, which have become scarily pertinent. Normalising of death in later life as 'natural' and expected (Howarth, 2007) has legitimised the neglect and inhumane treatment of older people at the end of their lives. Demonstrated by practices reported during the pandemic that contravene the human rights of older care home residents, such as blanket 'do not resuscitate' orders applied without the individuals' or their families' consent (AIUK, 2020, 2021; CQC, 2020; Stevenson, 2020; Wearmouth, 2020; Calvert and Arbuthnott, 2021). These issues along with other themes related to ageing and the crisis in health and social care are discussed further in the following chapter.

6

The COVID-19 health and social care challenge

Introduction

As Chapters 3 and 4 have argued, the challenges facing health and social care are the result of discursive and structural changes at the global and national level, namely globalisation, neoliberalisation and austerity. A shift from active to precarious ageing, alongside growing fragmentation, complexity, marketisation and intersecting inequalities, is illustrated in the empirical data in Chapter 5. The health and social care system have been in 'crisis' for many years; thus, the COVID-19 pandemic did not cause the 'crisis' in health and social care, but rather exacerbated it. Nevertheless, since COVID-19 hit in March 2020, the NHS has gone through the most challenging set of circumstances since its inception in 1948. Furthermore, it occurred at a time when health and social care institutions were underfunded, understaffed, fragmented and poorly coordinated with each other. The result of the pandemic was devastating for older people in the UK (particularly the tragedy of numerous deaths in care and residential homes) and this chapter provides an initial discussion of what went wrong. What follows is a comparative analysis of the respective COVID-19 health and social care policies of Sweden and Germany. Here, I revisit the two case studies detailed in Chapter 3, where Germany's and Sweden's health and social care systems were summarised. Finally, I discuss the impact of the COVID-19 and Brexit nexus on health and social care, and the ways forward the government is indicating it might take. Some of the policies offered by the Conservative government since taking power and securing a majority in 2015 related to integrating health and social care. These will also be critically examined considering the UK government's handling of the COVID-19 pandemic.

The impact of COVID-19 on the UK

Analysis of the empirical data in Chapter 5 has already established that health and social care services were not consistently providing good quality care or dignity to older people. Chapter 3 argued that neoliberalisation, together with the resulting privatisation of health and social care services, shifted responsibility for health and social care from the state to the individual, thereby re-establishing the very class inequalities that the welfare state was originally constructed to eradicate. This regressive reassertion of class inequalities has impacted health and social policy, exacerbating the precariousness of those most vulnerable. This is especially true for older women with low levels of capital. As a result of the underfunded, precarious systemic context produced by neoliberalism and privatisation, health and social care are susceptible to underperforming when any pressures are exerted on the system – for instance, austerity measures or a pandemic.

In March 2020, with nine months left in the final Brexit extension period, and the health and social care system already in crisis, the COVID-19 pandemic hit the UK with devastating effects (Horton, 2020). As stated in Chapter 4, since the economic crisis of 2008, austerity policies and associated cuts to public funds have eroded and undermined the ability of the health and social care system to provide good quality services to the public, particularly to vulnerable groups such as older people. COVID-19 exacerbated the challenges the UK's fragmented health and social care system already faced. The inequalities produced were laid bare by the high number of deaths. Those suffering the worst death rates were people over 80 years, older people living in residential settings, minority ethnic communities, those from working-class backgrounds, men and people working in care settings (usually women) (PHE, 2020; WBG, 2020). Apart from men, all these groups were already identified as being precarious within a marketised health and social care system. The groups hardest hit by the COVID-19 pandemic will be discussed in turn, starting with minority ethnic and working-class communities, followed by men and people working in care settings, and finishing with people over 80 years and older people living in residential settings.

Minority ethnic and working-class communities

When controlling for age, the highest death rates were among people from Black, Asian and mixed heritage backgrounds (Kirby, 2020; PHE, 2020; Platt and Warwick, 2020). There is a relationship between ethnicity, social class and geographical location (PHE, 2020) and, therefore, all these identities will be discussed together here. Unfortunately, the racialised disparity in COVID-19 deaths was predictable, given pre-existing and long-standing racialised health inequalities (Lawrence, 2020). Minority ethnic groups have always had lower life expectancies and poorer health and wellbeing outcomes compared with the White majority ethnic group in the UK, and these inequalities have only been exacerbated as a result of austerity and the neoliberal politics of class (Lawrence, 2020; see Chapter 3). Even in relation to access and the ability to implement public health information (such as COVID-19 health campaigns), social class and other intersecting inequalities have had an impact on the prevention of escalating health needs: 'People who struggle to access, understand, appraise and apply health information, or who face barriers in navigating the complexity of the NHS, may not be able to adhere to public health messages or advice' (PHE, 2020: 38; see Chapter 5).

These death rates are the result of entrenched structural racism and 'colour blindness', as well as the rescinding of the welfare state's commitments to the redistribution of wealth – a process which began with the Thatcherite politics of the 1980s and has continued through austerity and the anti-immigrant politics of Brexit Britain (Lawrence, 2020). The pandemic shone a light onto increasing disparities in access to education, social networks, occupational opportunities, housing, security, wealth and health – or as Bourdieu would call it, the possession of 'capital' (1984). If the UK is an 'arena of production', minority ethnic and working-class groups are struggling to invest and compete for resources (see Chapter 2). Bourdieu (1998) would also argue that this is a product of the denigration of the social and celebration of the economic, which has led to casualisation, flexibilisation and the erosion of social protections in the welfare state. This has disenfranchised workers and eradicated their ability to resist the undermining of their job security (Bourdieu, 1998). Globalisation has added another level of competition for scarce jobs, so workers now compete on a global scale, which further undermines working conditions, wages, security and their ability to resist (Bourdieu, 1998). People from minority ethnic backgrounds make up 21 per cent of NHS workers, but accounted for 63 per cent of NHS worker deaths (Razaq et al, 2020). The intersectionality of aged, minority ethnic and working-class identities have trebled the effects of inequalities of ageism, racism and classism (see Chapter 2). Those with the highest chances of dying from this virus are those who have been systematically discriminated against in society. For instance, the health of doctors from minority ethnic backgrounds is affected by racist practices in the NHS, where, for instance, twice as many minority ethnic as White doctors report being pressured to perform aerosol-generating procedures without adequate personal protective equipment (PPE) (BMA, 2020).

Men and health and social care workers

Men over the age of 65 years are twice as likely to die from COVID-19 than older women in the UK (PHE, 2020). It is not known definitively why men are more likely to die of the virus, but there are a number of factors that may explain the difference. These include differences in men's social behaviours (which may impact how they acquire the virus), as well as differences in how they understand symptoms and access care. Other explanations include gendered differences in immune responses and a higher prevalence of particular chronic illnesses caused by social behaviours like smoking and drinking (PHE, 2020; WBG, 2020). However, there are key worker jobs which men are predominately doing, for example, paramedics are 'key workers' doing precarious work in the COVID-19 pandemic (Campbell and Price, 2016). Paramedics have had high rates of transmission and unions have blamed the levels of PPE being inadequate (GMB, 2020), potentially putting older patients, who paramedics often attend to, at high risk of infection (see Chapter 5). Nevertheless, women are more likely to be employed in high-risk, low-paid roles (WBG, 2020), doing precarious work in precarious forms of employment (Vosko et al, 2009; Vosko, 2010; Standing, 2011; Campbell and Price, 2016; see Chapter 2). Women in precarious employment have few benefits, such as sickness pay, holiday pay or secure contracts (WBG, 2020). Women, therefore, have less economic capital than men and have been hit harder by the financial implications of COVID-19 and lockdowns (WBG, 2020). Notwithstanding higher rates of poverty, women have also experienced higher rates of domestic violence and have been required to provide disproportionate levels of unpaid care during the pandemic (WBG, 2020).

Women are exposed to precarious work in health and social care roles (Standing, 2011; Campbell and Price, 2016), especially during a pandemic. Furthermore, the PPE provided in health care settings often does not fit women well, because it has been designed for men. This puts women at a higher risk of infection (WBG, 2020). In domiciliary care, where the majority of workers are women, staff have reported having to buy their own PPE, as none has been provided by their organisations. This not only puts the care workers at risk, but also the mostly older people that they care for (UNISON, 2020), possibly accounting for the high rates of excess deaths of older people receiving domiciliary care in their own homes (see Hodgson et al, 2020). Finally, there has been no increase in the caring allowance for those providing unpaid care for older people (often spouses), despite the increase in caring activities, the rise in food costs and the lack of available respite during the pandemic (Carers UK, 2020a; WBG, 2020). As is clear, women in both paid and unpaid caring roles have been put at significantly greater risk during the pandemic, and their economic and mental wellbeing has suffered (Carers UK, 2020b; WBG, 2020).

Do older lives matter? Deaths of people over 80 and older people in residential settings

According to Public Health England (PHE) (2020), 75 per cent of deaths in the first wave of COVID-19 were people over 75 years old. However, the percentage of excess deaths was lower in the oldest age group (over 80 years) than other age groups (PHE, 2020). Therefore, although more older people died of COVID-19, a larger proportion of deaths in the oldest age category were not linked to COVID-19 compared with other age groups. This could be due to the lack of testing available in residential settings during the first wave, where more of the older age groups reside. It could also be attributed to the probability of death from any cause increasing with age, as does the presence of a chronic illness (Baltes and Mayer, 1999). However, this does not mean that chronic illnesses and vulnerability to COVID-19 is inevitable in later life; it just means it is more likely than in younger age groups. This is why the initial policy decision taken by the government to 'shield' all people over 65 years old was age-reductionist: calculating people's risk of contracting COVID-19 based only on chronological age is flawed and ageist (BSG, 2020). Nevertheless, the sequestration of people in residential care settings has been a characteristic of the inhumane treatment of mostly older people in the UK. With restricted visits from friends and family, older people's mental, physical and emotional wellbeing has been significantly affected (Age UK, 2020).

In fact, several different discourses of ageing informed policies and institutional responses to the pandemic in parallel. However, one of the more disturbing developments – and arguably an extreme example of biopolitical power (Foucault, 1978; see Chapter 2) – has been the UK government's intermittent use of a 'herd immunity' discourse, based on a logic that those most vulnerable to the virus (including older people and those with chronic health conditions) must be sacrificed for the immunity and wellbeing of the healthy younger population (Buffel et al, 2020; Horton, 2020; Calvert and Arbuthnott, 2021). Unlike biopower, however, this form of population management was not subtle and instead could be understood as a form of 'necropolitics', which is when state power implements modes of exception to decide who lives and who dies (Foucault, 1978; Mbembe, 2003; Robertson and Travaglia, 2020). Robertson and Travagia (2020) have applied the term necropolitics to the treatment of older people during the COVID-19 pandemic. Parallels can be seen in Mbmebe's (2003) writing, when discussing the spatialised control of populations who are at the whim of state decisions over their life and death, much like the older people in residential settings during the COVID-19 pandemic. Arguably, residential care settings and some hospital wards during the COVID-19 pandemic could be compared to 'death-worlds … in which vast populations are subjected to conditions of life conferring upon them the status of living dead' (Mbmebe, 2003: 40). This will be discussed further below in relation to some of the (exceptional) practices implemented during the COVID-19 pandemic, including, unsafe hospital discharges, denial of medical treatment and blanket 'Do Not Resuscitate' orders.

Unsafe hospital discharge

Although the government policy of herd immunity was initially dropped (albeit arguably reapplied over the summer of 2021 with the relaxation of all public health measures which prevented the spread of the virus), the invisible and lonely deaths of older people in care homes were implicitly condoned by society (Calvert and Arbuthnott, 2021). 'Care homes' experience has been far from being better protected and "having arms wrapped around them"; they were actually silenced, put out of sight and out of mind' (Stevenson, 2020: 226). The government claimed to not realise the implications of discharging older people who were symptomatic and asymptomatic from hospitals back to care homes, the evidence was there plain to see in March 2020, when in Madrid, Spain, it was estimated that 2,000 older care home residents died after the transmission of the virus in these settings took hold (AIUK, 2020; Horton, 2020; Phillipson, 2020b). Prior to COVID-19, it is well known in the literature that unsafe discharges were attributed to a number of factors, including not being clinically ready, not being assessed or consulted, relatives not being told about the discharge and patients being discharged with no care package in place (Glasby, 2003; Parliamentary and Health Service Ombudsman, 2016). Discharge from hospital is considered the most vulnerable point in the patient journey, involving many threats to patient safety, such as falls, incomplete testing, lack of ongoing care and risk of infection (Laugaland et al, 2012; Philibert and Barach, 2012; Waring et al, 2015). Furthermore, unsafe discharges can result in anxiety, deterioration of health, readmission to hospital and death (The Patients Association, 2020). A lack of information about ongoing care or medications is also reported by patients to be a problem (CQC, 2019). Although most clinicians recognise the importance of discharging patients safely, successful discharge planning and care transition depend upon the coordination of care in a fragmented health service; public, private and third-sector organisations need to work within and across organisational boundaries (Waring et al, 2015). Therefore, to expect residential care services to coordinate safety procedures in the first wave without any government guidance (which was not available until May 2020 [DHSC, 2020]), when the market was as fragmented and asset-stripped as it was (see Chapter 3), was naive at best, and negligent and callous at worst (Horton, 2020; Calvert and Arbuthnott, 2021).

Furthermore, Amnesty International UK (2020) reported that care home managers were pressurised to take residents who had not been tested or had tested positive for COVID-19, even though half of care home managers in May 2020 reported not having sufficient facilities to quarantine. Some even reported having older patients being dropped off at care homes in the middle of the night, to avoid their being refused admission, because a manager would not be there (AIUK, 2020). Other care homes in Durham reported being offered a 10 per cent increase in funding to take older people with unknown infection status (AIUK, 2020). Moreover, some families reported not being involved in the discharge decision-making process, rushing the older vulnerable person out of hospital sometimes even without their teeth or glasses (AIUK, 2020). This lack of involvement in decision-making regarding family members' care and end of life has been reported by research collecting experiences of bereavement during the pandemic (Harrop et al, 2020). Knowledge about patients gathered from family and their informal support is vital to ensure successful hospital discharge and continuity of care. Subsequent protocols regarding testing for COVID-19 when discharging older people from hospital did improve from 18 September 2020, with the inclusion of the requirement to test for COVID-19 and share the results with the care home prior to discharge (Healthwatch and British Red Cross, 2020).

Denial of medical treatment

However, unsafe discharges from hospital were unfortunately one of many neglectful and ageist practices towards older people during the COVID-19 pandemic. In care homes, managers reported being under pressure not to admit older people to hospital for care and in some cases, admission to hospital was refused even when that older person needed urgent care (AIUK, 2020). According to Calvert and Arbuthnott (2021: 203) in March 2020, health authorities justifying the exclusion of older people based on the assumption that being in hospital would not be beneficial. In some cases, GPs also refused to treat older residents in residential settings, which led to unqualified care home staff doing medical procedures and some older people dying in pain (AIUK, 2020). Furthermore, generally clinicians state that hospitals are seen as 'safe places' where older people can reside when they have nowhere else to go, which usually contrasts with their own view that hospitals are 'dangerous' places for older people to stay. This became appallingly accurate during the first wave of the COVID-19 pandemic in the UK, when the government's senior clinical advisors developed the 'COVID-19 triage score: sum of 3 domains' to ensure scenes broadcast on news programmes did not replicate those of Italian hospitals being overrun (Calvert and Arbuthnott, 2021: 211).

> It provided doctors with a framework for determining which patients should be selected for critical care based on three indicators: age, frailty and underlying conditions. Since any total over eight meant a patient would be given ward-based treatment only, the over 80s were automatically excluded because they were allocated a score of nine points for their age alone. It meant that age group would not be given intensive care. (Calvert and Arbuthnott, 2021: 228)

This proposed application of 'frailty' discourse, intended to categorise, biomedicalise, and subjectify older people in 'deep old age' to justify rationing life-saving treatment in the context of a health and social care system with 'precarious resources' (Grenier et al, 2017a, 2017b, 2020a; see Chapter 2). After subsequent revision, marks were lowered for age but raised for some underlying conditions, but still meant that people were denied critical care beds based on age at the peak of the first wave, when data suggests that with treatment, they would have had a four in ten chance of survival (Calvert and Arbuthnott, 2021). Although the guidance was formally withdrawn, it was distributed to clinicians around the UK, who claim they were forced to use it or something similar to the 'government-commissioned age-based "triage tool"' (Calvert and Arbuthnott, 2021: 229). In some cases, this rationing of life-saving treatment was being applied even when capacity was available; older patients were rigorously being confined to what one family member described as the 'death ward':

> Vivien says that inside there were eight elderly men infected with the virus whom she describes as the 'living dead'… lying 'half naked in nappies' on their beds in stifling heat looking 'drugged and dazed'. The scene was heart-breaking: 'To see people just dying, all around you'. (Calvert and Arbuthnott, 2021: 245)

Over 50 per cent of the people who died in hospitals during the first wave were over 80 years old, however only 2.5 per cent of patients over 80 were admitted to intensive care units and thus were denied lifesaving treatment (Calvert and Arbuthnott, 2021: 251). These kinds of illegal practices that contravene the UK Human Rights Act 1998, Article 2: the right to life are further examples of how older people in these spaces can be seen to inhabit 'death worlds' where spatialised control of populations are at the whim of state decisions over their life and death (Mbmebe, 2003: 40). In the cases uncovered by Amnesty International UK (2020) and Calvert and Arbuthnott (2021), older people in these exceptional state conditions have been marked as being worth less, and allowed to suffer and die in pain. The underfunded and fragmented health and social care system arguably reduced older people at one of the most vulnerable, precarious moments of their lives to 'bare life' (Agamben, 2005; Waring and Bishop, 2020). Older people's lives in the health and social care system have been devalued, legitimising poor treatment and undignified care (Waring and Bishop, 2020). Waring and Bishop (2020) and Agamben (2005) argue that Foucault's (1978) concept of biopower (see Chapter 2) is relevant to the production of deserving or underserving citizens in political–judicial systems. Hospitals have been designed to categorise people's bodies into discrete siloed departmental categories: respiratory equals lungs, orthopaedics equals bones and so on.

This means that older people's bodies do not fit (Humphries et al, 2016, see Chapter 2).

Considerable harm has also been inflicted on older people in domestic settings, especially when people have been asked to shield from the COVID-19 virus by not leaving their homes for months at a time (Age UK, 2020). Furthermore, in the UK, there were 4,500 excess deaths of older people receiving domiciliary care by July 2020, an increase of 225 per cent (Hodgson et al, 2020). It is unclear whether this is due to undiagnosed cases of COVID-19 or indirect impacts of not having access to health care, as many death certificates do not attribute COVID-19 as the cause (Hodgson et al, 2020). It is a complex picture because, like the residential care sector, the domiciliary sector is also mainly run by for-profit organisations, with underpaid and under-resourced staff (see Chapter 3). A particular challenge was providing access to adequate PPE and education around infection control procedures. Nevertheless, due to the lack of testing in people's own homes during the first wave, excess deaths is the only indicator of the number of people who might have died from COVID-19 at home without being conveyed to hospital. According to Calvert and Arbuthnott (2021: 263), there were 25,200 excess deaths in England and Wales in the first six months of the pandemic. Ambulance services were directed to exclude 'elderly' patients, both those in their own homes and residential care settings (Calvert and Arbuthnott, 2021).

> A paramedic in London said he would normally be 'in and out of care homes all the time' attending to emergencies. 'We'd typically go in twice a week', he said. 'But I didn't attend a single care home from the beginning of April to the end of April during that first peak.' (Calvert and Arbuthnott, 2021: 283)

Accounts of older people being denied access to hospital care in the first wave by paramedic services were reported to the CQC (2021) and multiple reports of care home residents not being conveyed to hospital are also detailed in a report by Amnesty International UK (2020).

Blanket 'Do Not Resuscitate' orders

This denial of access to treatment is further compounded if older people have limited economic, social or cultural capital, and lack families and friends to advocate on their behalf (see Chapter 5). For instance, during the pandemic, end of life policies were distorted to deny older people the right to treatment, with reports of older people being pressured to sign do not resuscitate (DNR) forms, and of GPs and care homes being asked to encourage patients to waive their right to treatment (AIUK,

2020, 2021; CQC, 2020, 2021; Stevenson, 2020; Wearmouth, 2020; Calvert and Arbuthnott, 2021). Further, the CQC (2021) has reported a significant increase in DNR orders for people in residential care during the pandemic (March–December 2020) and some could contravene human rights legislation.

> A DNR is a legal order indicating that a person does not want invasive intervention to prevent them dying. This requires sensitive discussions with a person about their wishes towards the end of their life and can be designed to empower frail older and disabled people. However, instructions were given to some care home managers to apply DNRs to all residents. Ignoring the individual's wishes and medical condition is to blatantly contravene the Human Rights Act 1998, Article 2: the right to life. (Stevenson, 2020: 221)

As discussed in Chapter 5, clinicians reported that sensitive end of life conversations require long-standing, trusting relationships with patients alongside their families, and these discussions need to take place in quiet and calm environments, preferably not in a busy hospital setting. However, during the pandemic, Amnesty International UK (2020) found that families and patients were asked to sign DNR forms without understanding what they meant (see Chapter 5 for discussion of cognitive capital in emergency situations). Furthermore, in March 2020, a document was issued by the Sussex Clinical Commissioning Group (CCG) to GPs, asking them to find and issue DNRs to care home residents without the orders (AIUK, 2020). Following a media outcry, this guidance was quickly retracted, but Sussex was not the only CCG to do this, as it was reported that the directive came from above (AIUK, 2020). Furthermore, relatives of people who died in residential and hospital settings were not able to see or say goodbye to their loved ones in a way they would have liked; in some cases experiencing distressing and traumatic experiences such as listening to their relatives die over the telephone (Harrop et al, 2020).

It is undeniable that the treatment of older people in hospital and residential settings, including their subsequent quarantining from friends and family, has been abhorrent. It began with high death rates in the first wave, when in the UK at the end of May 2020, 46,000 people had died of COVID-19 in England and Wales; four out of five of them were aged 70 or over (Webb, 2020). During the first wave of the pandemic (mid–March to end of June 2020), 31 per cent of all registered deaths in the UK were in care homes (Bell et al, 2020). The fragmentation in the health and social care system across the UK is even observable in death registration and testing practices, thus this made it difficult to analyse COVID-19 deaths in care homes; which is why Bell et al (2020) also used excess deaths in their analysis. English care homes reported the highest increase in excess deaths (79 per cent), followed by a 62 per cent increase in Scottish, 66 per cent in Welsh and 46 per cent in Northern Irish care homes (Bell et al, 2020). Data on transfers of care to and from hospital to residential settings were also unreliable, as were data reporting testing practices for residents and staff, due to turbulent access to tests in the first wave (Bell et al, 2020). The King's Fund's analysis of this tragedy was as follows:

> Despite the best efforts of staff, it has been difficult for care providers to keep staff and people relying on services safe. A variety of factors contributed to this, including: challenges obtaining adequate PPE, testing and financial support; difficulties in co-ordinating the response across a fragmented sector; longer-term weaknesses resulting from years of under-investment and workforce shortages; and rapid discharges from hospitals to care homes early in the pandemic. Despite strong international evidence that social care settings were at high risk from serious infection, the sector was treated as an afterthought by government at the start of the pandemic, with support measures coming too little and too late. (Charles and Ewbank, 2020)

More importantly, in the first wave, the systematic denial of treatment and right to life based on ageism and the application of biomedical discourses of frailty to deep old age in hospitals, residential care settings and people's own homes led to the unnecessary deaths of thousands of older people (see above, Grenier et al, 2017a, 2017b, 2020b; AIUK, 2020, 2021; CQC, 2020, 2021; Stevenson, 2020; Wearmouth, 2020; Calvert and Arbuthnott, 2021).

Negligence and the second wave

In the UK, the second wave of the COVID-19 pandemic followed a summer where infection rates were low, so in August 2020, the government encouraged the UK population to 'eat out to help out' the economy. Restaurant meals had reduced by 50 per cent and, at the time, it's been estimated that this economic policy accounted for 8–17 per cent of COVID-19 cases (Fetzer, 2020). Furthermore, conceptualising the economy and health as being mutually exclusive was presented as a false economy, and this acted to shorten the time between the end of the first wave and the beginning of the second (Fetzer, 2020). Concurrently, a series of failures by autumn with regard to the 'NHS track and trace' system – run by Conservative Peer Dido Harding and outsourced to private companies including Serco and Sitel – (Mazzucato, 2021), according to the Scientific Group for Emergencies (SAGE), was only having a 'marginal impact' on stopping the spread of COVID-19 (Volpicelli, 2020: n.p.).

Additionally, over sucessive summers, warnings grew regarding the impact that sending school pupils and university students back to in-person classes would have on infection rates in the surrounding communities. For example, in August 2020, the University and College Union warned this would spark a second wave of infections with students trapped in residence halls (UCU, 2020). The government and universities (which are independent third-sector marketised organisations) ignored these predictions and, in October, infection rates at universities rose to seven times higher than in the surrounding areas and students were imprisoned in their rooms (McIntyre et al, 2020). Following this, the tier systems brought in by England's government to provide regionally targeted responses proved woefully inadequate against a virus that could travel across regional (and national) boundaries via people's bodies (Calvert and Arbuthnott, 2021). SAGE advised the UK government to administer a 'circuit-breaker' lockdown in early October, which was rejected for being too damaging to the economy (James, 2020; Calvert and Arbuthnott, 2021), until cases soared and a second month-long UK-wide lockdown was announced at the end of October 2020 (spanning 5 November – 2 December 2020).

In early December 2020, the impact of a new variant of COVID-19 (first identified in Kent on 20 September 2020) was discussed in PHE. Cases of the variant had increased in November during the second lockdown (Mahase, 2020). On 24 November, the government announced the loosening of COVID-19 rules for the five days over Christmas (Murray, 2020), instructing individuals to take 'personal responsibility' for the spread of COVID-19 (Cabinet Office, 2020). This policy was maintained in December, despite SAGE advisors, epidemiologists and doctors warning that relaxing the rules at the height of a pandemic, on top of winter pressures on the NHS was 'kamikaze' and would lead to unnecessary deaths (Davis, 2020). Finally, on 18 December 2020, the Prime Minister changed the Christmas relaxation plans, but mainly focussed on tough restrictions in the South East, where the new variant was then clustered (Mahase, 2020). As predicted, over Christmas 2020, rates of infections, hospitalisations and deaths increased rapidly. The UK then went into its third national lockdown on 4 January 2021 (Cabinet Office, 2021). Unfortunately, this catalogue of failures, delays and policies relaxing safety measures to prioritise the economy has come at the expense of (older) people's lives (Calvert and Arbuthnott, 2021). In mid-January 2021, the UK had one of the worst COVID-19 death rates in the world, with over 100,000 having died within 28 days of testing positive for COVID-19 (Barr et al, 2021). Even with a successful vaccination programme that administered two doses to 72 per cent of over 18s in England within nine months (NHS England, 2021), by 9 August 2021, the UK still had the 18th worst death rate in the world, with 1,945 dead per million people (de Best, 2021).

Neoliberalism, intergenerational conflict and 'new ageism'

It hasn't just been the British government that considered the lives of thousands of older people a price worth paying for the economy; the complete disregard for the lives of older people has also been replicated elsewhere in the world. In the US, for instance, a Texan politician referred to the pandemic as the 'Boomer remover', suggesting that grandparents should be sacrificed for the sake of the economy (Calasanti, 2020b). This argument is based on a lethal mixture of biomedical and economic reductionist ageing narratives (see Chapter 2). It constructs people in later life as economically unproductive bodies that are a burden and drain on society (Calasanti, 2020a). This 'intergenerational conflict' narrative is particularly popular in neoliberal politics, where a commitment to the reduction in the welfare state finds a convenient target in older people (Carney and Nash, 2020). The myth that older people's wellbeing is at odds with younger people's is easily undermined by taking a long-term view; if older people's lives and welfare are eroded, then the same will happen to future generations, if lucky enough to reach old age (Carney and Nash, 2020). However, by using this argument, the state avoids paying higher welfare bills (Carney and Nash, 2020). This analysis can be neatly applied to the COVID-19 pandemic. 'New ageism', a term coined by Walker (2012), has been used to encapsulate the divisive political rhetoric that pitches one generation against another. It is the argument older people have too many rights and benefits, and this inequity is harming younger people (Carney and Nash, 2020). During the COVID-19 pandemic, neoliberal rhetoric has been successful in perpetuating new ageism by arguing that older lives are worth less than younger lives. Therefore, the UK's response has arguably been shaped by its neoliberal/Anglo–Saxon modelling (Esping-Andersen, 1990, see Chapter 3), but how did the other welfare state models fare under the stresses of the COVID-19 pandemic?

Comparative contemporary analysis of Sweden's and Germany's handling of COVID-19

As discussed in Chapter 3, Sweden, Germany and the UK are seen as archetypal examples of three very different welfare state models: the social–democratic/ Scandinavian model, the corporatist/Continental European model, and the neoliberal/Anglo–Saxon model, respectively (Esping-Andersen, 1990, see Chapter 3). The three countries have responded differently to COVID-19, and this section will outline the policies implemented by the Swedish and German governments in order to compare these with each other and with those of the UK government. This section will recap each country's health and social care system and then examine how these different configurations performed in response to the first wave of the pandemic, with a particular focus on the health and social care provided to older people. The aim of this section is to establish whether the UK can learn anything from the other two countries about its health and social care system, and its handling of the COVID-19 pandemic.

Sweden: herd immunity

As part of a social-democratic model of the welfare state, Sweden has historically been known for strong welfare policies of various kinds. However, even Sweden's health and social care services have been increasingly marketised, with the outsourcing of key services to large multinational conglomerates making lucrative profits (Anttonen and Karsio, 2017). These have been critiqued for introducing new costs into the system, with private providers cherry-picking lucrative patients (Anttonen and Karsio, 2017). In 2016, around a quarter of home care services and residential care homes were privately run and suffering from fragmentation, complex governance structures, and a lack of accountability and accessibility (Anttonen and Karsio, 2017). Since the 1990 reforms, fewer people in later life receive social and health care in their homes (Sundstrom and Tortosa, 1999; Anderson and Karlberg, 2000). Furthermore, staffing in residential care settings has been significantly reduced, with many working on hourly contracts and with low competency levels (Stolt et al, 2011). In 2011, Triton, the largest for-profit organisation in the field, was involved in a media scandal for providing poor-quality care and having high death rates among older residents. It was subsequently restructured, rebranded and broken up into Vardaga and Ambea (Harrington et al, 2017). Some argue that Sweden's welfare policies have more broadly shifted from an egalitarian ideal of equality of outcome to ideals of choice and diversity, delivered via privatisation (Meagher and Szebehely, 2019). Nevertheless, the Swedish government was still largely seen as competent at governing these new markets, and older people's health and social care services are still publicly funded (Anttonen and Karsio, 2017).

Interestingly, like the UK, which also has a social care market that is largely privatised, Sweden started its response to COVID-19 with a herd immunity policy. However, following an Imperial College London study that predicted half a million deaths in the UK if its government continued with minimal intervention, the UK government appeared to change tack, but the Swedish government explicitly continued to follow this policy (Karlsson, 2020). Anders Tegnell, Sweden's state epidemiologist, defended his 'light touch strategy', which only implemented a ban on visitors to residential homes, and did not issue guidance on infection control and use of PPE until 1 April 2020. This led to three times as many deaths per million residents as in Denmark in the first wave, Scandinavia's second worst-hit country (Karlsson, 2020). Older people were not protected in domiciliary and residential home settings and, by 1 June 2020, 62 per cent of deaths were of people over 70 years in residential settings or at home receiving domiciliary care (Karlsson, 2020). A lockdown would have provided Sweden time to get testing and tracing up and running (which it was slow to do), and would have helped to protect the most vulnerable (Karlsson, 2020).

Like in the UK, staff in private residential homes or providing domiciliary care in Sweden are low-paid, younger, often live in multi-occupancy households and take public transport to work. Therefore, the very people caring for those at the highest risk of death were at the highest risk of being infected by the virus and of spreading it to the older people for whom they were caring (Karlsson, 2020). The inadequate attempts at protecting older people in Sweden during this pandemic, however, must be situated within the wider neoliberalisation of its health and social care market. For instance, in 2017, residential homes were accused of under-investing to the point where understaffing and inadequate training led to older people being undernourished and, in 2018, 600 excess deaths were reported due to inadequate ventilation during a heat wave (Karlsson, 2020). During COVID-19, this trend of under-investment and negligence continued. In the first wave, staff at large conglomerate-owned residential homes reported a lack of PPE and unsafe quarantine practices whereby they were caring for healthy and infected residents concurrently; one home is under criminal investigation (Karlsson, 2020). Within the context of neoliberalism and the privatisation of services, politicians and private companies were able to blame each other and avoid accountability. Thus, it could be argued that Sweden prioritised its economy above the lives of its older generations, using narratives of personal responsibility and citizenship to justify its actions. Nevertheless, by the end of the first wave in June 2020, faced with this initial excessive death toll, the government promised an inquiry and committed 2.2 billion Swedish kronor towards training staff and providing resources for health and social care for older people (Karlsson, 2020).

The second wave of COVID-19 hit Sweden in the autumn of 2020 and the hope that herd immunity from the first wave would help to ease cases and deaths in the second did not pan out (Orange, 2020; Calvert and Arbuthnott; 2021). With increasing cases putting a strain on the health system and increasing numbers of health staff becoming infected, Sweden's government introduced a curfew on bars and a ban on meeting in groups of more than eight (*The Guardian*, 2020). The inquiry set up after the first wave reported that the under-resourced and fragmented health and social care system for older people was partly to blame for deaths in the first wave, alongside insufficient and late restrictions being implemented by the Swedish government (*The Guardian*, 2020; Calvert and Arbuthnott; 2021). In December 2020, failures to shield and treat the most vulnerable older people was heavily criticised by Sweden's health and social care inspectorate, as reports claimed that fewer than one in 20 older people in residential settings had physically seen a doctor, with many regions issuing blanket bans on older people being treated in hospital and some doctors prescribing end of life care for older residents without sight of their medical notes (Orange, 2020). On 9 August 2021, Sweden had the worst death rate of all Nordic countries and the 24th worst in the world, with 1,425 deaths per million people, in comparision to 150 in Norway and 180 in Finland (de Best, 2021).

Germany: protect, track and trace

The German health system was founded on corporatist traditions, first establishing an insurance system in the late 19th century (Moran, 1999). Since the 1950s there has been a shift from health services being free at the point of contact to patients contributing to the costs of health care consumption (Moran, 1999). Following mass unemployment after reunification, markets and state regulation were introduced – both key characteristics of neoliberal politics (Moran, 1999), as are customer choice, competitive tendering and pressure to derive profits from 'efficiency savings' (Moran, 1999). From 1994, all older people (as well as the rest of the population) were insured for health and social care costs (Busse and Riesberg, 2004). However, the health insurance reforms of the 1990s led to the marketisation of the residential and home–based care sector, although the dominance of charities providing residential care has largely continued (Bahle, 2003; Grohls et al, 2015). Due to the decentralised political and financial structure, the provision of end of life care has received criticism for being patchy or non–existent (Buser et al, 2008). As has involving older patients in end of life care discussions in hospitals (Jox et al 2010). Nevertheless, by law, older people have the right to choose whether care is provided by family, or by domiciliary, residential or ambulatory carers (Bahle, 2003).

When it came to responding to COVID-19, Germany's federal state system, with local health authority autonomy, swiftly implemented 'testing and tracing' systems, unlike the UK, which contracted out testing to an accounting firm (Reintjes, 2020; Mazzucato, 2021). Germany went into lockdown on 16 March 2020 and bans on residential care home visits were strictly enforced (Carroll et al, 2020). A two-week quarantine procedure was also strictly enforced for residents being discharged from hospital back into their residential homes. As a result of these measures, only 0.4 per cent of the older people in residential homes in Germany died from COVID-19 by 23 June 2020. In comparison, after the first wave of COVID-19, the UK rate was 13 times higher, at 5.2 per cent (Comas-Herrera et al, 2020). Discrimination against people based on age is prohibited in Germany, and this legal framework may lie behind the rigour with which residential homes and people receiving domiciliary care were protected (Comas-Herrera et al, 2020). Therefore, although Germany also provides some care to its older residents privately (although charity provision is still dominant), it had outlawed age discrimination legislatively and its local health authorities were able to respond quickly to protect older people during the first wave of the COVID-19 pandemic.

As the second wave of COVID-19 infections began to rise in the autumn of 2020, Germany's government introduced 'lockdown light' in November, but restrictions were quickly tightened (Sinclair, 2021). Shops and schools were closed throughout December 2020 and into January 2021, with a maximum of five people allowed to meet indoors (France, 2020). The national lockdown was extended until mid-February 2021, with new instructions to require higher-grade face masks on public transport and in shops, and employers instructed to allow people to work from home (Sinclair, 2021). Although Germany had challenges with its vaccination programme (due to administrative and cultural issues), with only 13.8 per cent of the population having received the first dose by 8 April, a change in strategy from mass vaccination centres to family doctor surgeries has increased the vaccination rate (*Metro US*, 2021). As of 2 August 2021, 52 per cent of the German population had received two doses of the vaccine (The Local, 2021). Notwithstanding the initial problematic vaccination strategy, Germany's death rate for COVID-19 as of 9 August was still significantly better then the UK, with 1,104 deaths per million people, putting it 45th in the world (de Best, 2021).

There are lessons that the UK government could have learnt from Germany in its handling of the first wave of the COVID-19 pandemic, particularly in relation to the legal protection of older people's right to health care and the implementation of track and trace to control the spread of the virus (Mazzucato, 2021). Yet, as described, the UK failed to implement these measures, and was slower to enact national lockdowns and implemented an inconsistent face mask wearing policy. However, the UK government also has another challenge to its precarious health and social care system: the aftermath of Brexit.

The COVID-19–Brexit nexus

The aftermath of COVID-19 and Brexit will almost certainly raise major issues for the future of health and social care in the UK. The pandemic has highlighted the weaknesses in the system and the deep inequalities that exist in society more generally (Charles and Ewbank, 2020). This includes the pressures on staffing and the growing numbers of vacancies that need to be filled (Charles and Ewbank, 2020; Tovey, 2020). This is notwithstanding the repercussions of the UK's exit from the European Union, which could include a rise in the cost of medicines, an increase in demand for care services (for returning emigrants) and ever-larger funding shortfalls (Murray et al, 2019). However, as Charles and Ewbank (2020) write:

... the [first] lockdown has caused deep damage to public finances and the wider economy. The social and economic consequences of the crisis, and the recession that is certain to follow, will undoubtedly have an impact on the population's health and mental wellbeing, and risk deepening inequalities further. (Charles and Ewbank, 2020)

In addition, the government is under pressure to revise the points-based immigration system, which does not make any allowances for social care workers, who are paid under £25,000 a year. This is likely to put off the majority of migrant workers in social care and some in the NHS, further exacerbating staff shortages.

Conservative policy post-COVID-19 and Brexit

In July 2020, during the COVID-19 crisis, Prime Minister Boris Johnson indicated that he wanted more control over the NHS, citing his frustration at having to persuade NHS Chief Executive Simon Stevens of what to do rather than simply tell him (Campbell, 2020). Greater political control would undo much of the last top-down reorganisation of the NHS in 2012 with the Health and Social Care Act and would reverse policy from competition to collaboration (Campbell, 2020; DHSC in Health Policy Insight, 2021). While the prospect of greater integration is welcomed by organisations like The King's Fund, another restructuring is not. As the implementation of the Health and Social Care Act demonstrated, restructuring tends to disrupt and distract staff from providing frontline services, and often has unwanted and unintended consequences (Charles and Ewbank, 2020). Particularly worrying is the prospect of the government 'taking back control' of the NHS, particularly following the disastrous management of the NHS track and trace system. The NHS has on the surface performed well despite the neoliberal measures imposed on it, such as funding shortages and the freezing of staff pay. It has also continued to perform during the COVID-19 pandemic, including in the subsequent waves, when it tried to continue with planned operations while rolling out a vaccination programme. This was despite the government's delays and inconsistencies in the provision of PPE, implementing social distancing, lockdown measures, face mask requirements and border restrictions, as well as having an inadequate track and trace system. The government has also announced the restructuring of PHE into two distinct bodies responsible for 'health security' and 'health improvement', both with greater political involvement (DHSC, 2021a, see Chapter 5). Concerns have been raised regarding the implications this political control will have on levels of transparency and accountability, but the intention to increase coherency at the local, regional, and national levels has been welcomed (Murray, 2021).

Improving integration or increasing privatisation?

As a result of the Health and Social Care Act 2012, which legislated for more competition, health and social care organisations have struggled to work together (see Chapter 3). The government has acknowledged that care for older people is inadequate and not fit for purpose; the fragmented and siloed nature of health and social care needs to be broken down, and services need to work collaboratively to deliver better-quality care (DHSC in Health Policy Insight, 2021). The introduction of new models of care began in 2015, with a number of variants, including the moving of specialist care services into the community (known as multispecialty community providers or MCPs), and the joining up of all health care organisations, such as GPs, mental health services, community services and hospitals into primary and acute care systems (PACSs) (NHS England, 2017). These integrated systems covered a population of five million people and worked together to reduce hospital admissions and the use of emergency inpatient day beds (NHS England, 2017). Sustainability and transformation partnerships (STPs) were then implemented across the UK as voluntary collaborations among health care providers to deliver health care tailored to the needs of local populations (NHS England, 2017). A more controversial element of this policy was the introduction of accountable care organisations (ACOs). ACOs, which originated in the US, are organisations that manage the costs associated with the care of a local population (Ham and Charles, 2018). The concern was this would lead to more private organisations being commissioned to deliver health and care services (Ham and Charles, 2018). Another concern was that the implementation of these organisations, alongside Brexit and trade deals with the United States, would lead to US organisations providing health care in the UK (Ham and Charles, 2018). As a result of two judicial reviews against NHS England in regard to ACOs, the name was changed. 'The NHS long term plan' (NHS England, 2019) set out that these contracts would likely be made with the now-rebranded integrated care systems (ICSs) (Charles, 2020). Although these new ways of delivering health and social care look promising, a number of criticisms have been levelled at them, including a lack of transparency, unrealistic financial savings and hospital admission targets, and a lack of involvement with the community (Charles, 2020).

In February 2021, a policy paper entitled 'Integration and innovation: working together to improve health and social care for all' (DHSC, 2021b) proposed putting ICSs into statute, with a legal 'duty of collaboration' instead of enforcing competitive tendering and replacing the CCGs' commissioning functions (Health Policy Insight, 2021). While effectively reversing Langley's controversial Health and Social Care Act 2012 is welcome (see Chapter 4), the overall control of the NHS (including ICSs and NHS England) passing to the Secretary of State for Health and Social Care, who would have the potential to intervene in the delivery of local health services, is concerning

(McKenna, 2021), particularly considering the management of NHS track and trace via outsourced private companies discussed earlier in this chapter. Furthermore, the draft act does not address the deep-rooted inequalities within the system, the urgent need to reform social care or chronic workforce shortages (Health Policy Insight, 2021; McKenna, 2021). Thus, it remains to be seen whether this proposed legislation will lead to cultural change and the innovative solutions needed to heal the damage already done to the health and social care system in the UK by austerity, COVID-19 and Brexit.

Conclusion

Unfortunately, the high death rates of older people in care homes as a result of COVID-19 in the UK is not surprising given the highly privatised residential home sector, which has little or no accountability to the highly vulnerable service users whom they were supposed to be protecting. The challenges faced by the sector – financial pressures, workforce shortages, the unsustainability of residential care markets – have been well-documented and are a product of decades of neoliberal policy and, more recently, austerity measures. When the COVID-19 pandemic hit in the spring of 2020, the health and social care system was already in crisis and, with a government that was willing to sacrifice its older population for the sake of the economy, the outlook was not rosy. The lockdown measures in the first (and subsequent) waves were too slow to prevent the spread of COVID-19 in the community (Horton, 2020). Residential care homes were not managed by the government and, in the first wave, did not provide adequate PPE, and the NHS discharged infectious older people to care homes without testing or quarantining measures (AIUK, 2020). Similarly, private organisations running domiciliary care services did not adequately protect their staff or older vulnerable service users in the first wave. Most importantly, the systematic denial of treatment and right to life based on ageism and the application of biomedical discourses of frailty to deep old age in hospitals, residential care settings and people's own homes led to the unnecessary deaths of thousands of older people (Grenier et al, 2017a, 2017b, 2020b; AIUK, 2020, 2021; CQC, 2020, 2021; Stevenson, 2020; Wearmouth, 2020; Calvert and Arbuthnott, 2021). Then a catalogue of neoliberal policy failures, which treated the economy and health as mutually exclusive (Calvert and Arbuthnott, 2021), led to subsequent waves, which proved more deadly than the first. Older people's lives have been sacrificed and this has been justified through new ageism, by propagating myths regarding intergenerational conflict, as well as biologically and economically reductionist discourses that construct older life as being worth less. The intersectionality of inequalities has also been laid bare, with people from minority ethnic and working-class communities dying in greater numbers. More men than women have died, but women working in health and social care roles have been exposed to higher risks of infection. The impact on the wider community of entire cohorts and generations of families dying will be significant.

Despite being held up as a model social-democratic country, Sweden also failed its older population and, like the UK, demonstrated a blatant disregard for their lives by failing to shield and/or treat, with accounts of malpractice in relation to end of life care. Sweden's under-resourced and fragmented health and social care system for older people was blamed, along with insufficient and late restrictions. Germany's health and social care system fared much better, with its locally organised and devolved federal system. There were lessons that the UK government could have learnt from Germany in its handling of the first wave of the COVID-19 pandemic, particularly in relation to the legal protection of older people's right to health care and the implementation of track and trace to control the spread of the virus. Yet, as described, the UK failed at implementing these measures and has been slower to enact national lockdowns and requirements to wear face masks.

In the aftermath of COVID-19 and Brexit, a recession is likely to extend beyond 2021. The government needs to acknowledge its policy failings and act fast to address the gaping holes in the health and social care system, particularly in relation to workforce shortages. However, Johnson's government has consistently deflected blame, accountability and responsibility for the pandemic, to individuals (those tasked with 'staying alert' against the virus) (Dowding, 2020), to companies (tasked with ensuring 'COVID-safe' workplaces) (Anderson, 2020), the NHS (Campbell, 2020), residential care homes (Walker et al, 2020) and the UK COVID-19 variant (Stewart et al, 2021). Despite the shortcomings of this government in managing the pandemic using the private sector, Johnson has announced yet another restructure to 'take back control' of the publicly run NHS, instead of restructuring the mainly privately run social care market. Giving conservative politicians power over the local delivery of NHS services is concerning. Particularly when the priority should be a comprehensive restructuring of social care, ensuring all providers are not-for-profit so that funding can be reinvested into wages and training for frontline staff and services for the residents or service users, not giving greater powers to private companies within the NHS. The next and final chapter examines some alternative health and social care solutions that prioritise older people's care over profits, and have been trialled but not adopted fully in the UK. The chapter will also summarise the themes of this book.

7

Innovative solutions and cultural change

Neoliberal political discourses have become inculcated in British and other northern European cultures, to the extent that it is normal to assume that individuals are responsible for their health and wellbeing, regardless of the inequalities they may have faced based on their social class, gender or ethnic background. However, this ignores how structural advantages and disadvantages accumulate across the lifecourse, producing contrasting experiences in later life, including in relation to health outcomes and life expectancy (Van de Mheen et al, 1998). Healthism is a political response often used at times of crisis when governments wish to deflect blame onto individuals (Crawford, 1980). This is illustrated in the UK government's response to COVID-19, which has generally ignored the structural inequalities faced by older people (ageism), people from minority ethnic backgrounds (racism), people with 'dis'abilities (disablism) and people from working-class backgrounds (classism), and how these put them at greater risk of contracting and dying from the virus. Older people's lives have been systematically neglected in residential, domiciliary and hospital care (Horton, 2020; Calvert and Arbuthnott, 2021). Furthermore, people from minority ethnic and working-class backgrounds have also been systemically disadvantaged and discriminated against in their workplaces and everyday lives (Lawrence, 2020). The intersectionality of inequalities has been demonstrated in the high death rates within these groups during the pandemic. However, these inequalities are far from new. Those with less economic, social, cultural, physical and cognitive capital have always had worse outcomes in health and social care systems, and these inequalities have been deepening in the UK since the 1980s.

Globalisation and neoliberalism need to be challenged. Governments and nation-states have a choice about whether to adopt policies that exacerbate inequalities and whether to outsource publicly run and financed services. Although globalisation and neoliberalism have been conceptualised as two entrenched yet resurgent systems of class and racial inequality, in the context of post or late modernity, developments in finance and information technology have occurred at a speed and breadth never seen before (Beck, 1999). Neoliberalism has been used to re-establish elite class power; however, like all discourses, it has changed over time (Mirowski, 2013). Proponents of neoliberalism have repealed policies that sought to progressively redistribute wealth and power to the working classes (the welfare state), with the aim of re-establishing class power via market elites, enforcing these new powers through regulation (Harvey, 2005). Nevertheless, all discourses can shift, be rejected and be replaced by alternatives. This concluding chapter considers alternatives to the outsourcing of care homes to multinational conglomerates that siphon off public funds and place them in the hands of shareholders. Moreover, the chapter considers whether there are better models for delivering domiciliary care – ones that are inexpensive but still provide quality care and adequate wages for staff.

Although Boris Johnson used Churchillian rhetoric during the first wave of the COVID-19 pandemic to convey a sense of fighting a war against the virus (Hamad, 2020; Horton; 2020), like Churchill himself during the London smog of 1952, Johnson ignored the structural impact of systemic policies that put the economy above the health of those most precarious in society, resulting in the death of thousands of innocent people. In fact, much like Churchill, who attributed the London smog of 1952 to the weather rather than to air pollution (Brimblecombe, 1987), Johnson trivialised COVID-19 in the early stages, shaking the hands of infected patients, ignoring the advice of his own scientific advisors and subsequently contracting the virus himself (Mason, 2020). In fact, it was only after contracting the virus that Johnson publicly praised NHS staff, thanking the doctors and nurses (mostly from minority ethnic backgrounds) who had treated him in London. This display of support was considered hypocritical by many, given the decade of frozen public-sector pay, which Johnson had voted for, as well as Johnson's role in engineering Brexit, which will result in thousands of doctors and nurses from the EU leaving the NHS (Hamad, 2020). Furthermore, the hypocrisy of Johnson presenting himself as pro-NHS by joining the UK public's demonstrations of thanks, clapping for carers (see https://clapforourcarers. co.uk/) or giving NHS workers a badge as a token of appreciation is blatant (BBC, 2020). Even with a pay increase above inflation for doctors in England (although, controversially, not social or other health care workers), they are still not paid the equivalent of pre-austerity policy levels in 2010 (BBC, 2020).

Although this book shows individual experiences of older people and health care workers before the pandemic, the case studies – in public health, pre-emergency, and end of life care settings – demonstrate the shift towards and the growing amplification of precarity experienced as a result of global discourses and national-level policy. Thus, the global-, national- and individual-level analysis has demonstrated how discourse and structure shape the lives of individuals. COVID-19 has just shone a very bright light on these same mechanisms and the devastating effects they produce. However, this pandemic could also provide an opportunity for change and reimagining. Thus, the rest of this chapter discusses alternative innovative solutions to the crisis in the health and social care system, and models that have already been trialled in the UK. Finally, this book ends with a consideration of what I argue are key issues of cultural change, necessary for better health and social care experiences for older people in the UK.

Innovative, alternative health and social care models

Over the years, many alternative innovative health and social care solutions have been trialled in the UK but not adopted fully. This section discusses what we can learn from some of these developments. The four that have been chosen as examples are the Homeshare scheme, therapeutic nursing homes, age-friendly cities and relational/asset-based approaches.

Homeshare: intergenerational support

Homeshare is a scheme that matches older people with a spare room in their houses with younger people who provide befriending and informal 'care' (Fox, 2018). Coffey (2010: 5) describes Homeshare as an arrangement whereby a person who requires some support in order to live independently can exchange accommodation for the support. Accommodation in the form of a spare room is offered in exchange for ten hours of support each week (Coffey, 2010: 5).

Previous research has found that this scheme benefits both parties and most matches were sustained for several months (Coffey, 2010). This scheme could provide significant benefits both for individuals and society (by preventing poor health and isolation, as well as saving taxpayer money [Carstein, 2003]), but the main barrier to the service being commissioned by CCGs and receiving direct referrals from health care professionals is the perception of safety issues, even though safety concerns do not feature heavily in existing evaluations of the scheme (Bulmer, 2010; Coffey, 2010; Bazalgette and Salter, 2013; SharedLivesPlus, 2016). Friendship networks can help individuals be active informally. This, according to Rainey (1998), helps reduce people's sense of reliance on formal organisations and contributes to their sense of empowerment and of belonging to a community (Fast and de Jong Gierveld, 2008). However, inappropriate and poorly located housing often restricts older people's ability to socialise and thereby narrows their social circles (Bazalgette and Salter, 2013). Furthermore, some older people feel retirement housing is akin to living in 'age-segregated ghettos'; therefore, this type of age-exclusive housing needs to be questioned and challenged (Bazalgette and Salter, 2013). Benefits of the Homeshare scheme include increased confidence for both parties and improved understanding between participants of different generations. The scheme has also challenged negative ageist stereotypes (Bulmer, 2010).

Although popular in Europe and all over the world, there seems to be a cultural dimension as to why this scheme has not been adopted universally in the UK, which impacts on the hermeneutics of the home, but also on how institutions like CCGs manage risk (Fox, 2018). For example, British culture seems to find it unacceptable for non-family members to live together. Relationships of non-related people in the UK tend to be conceptualised through an economic frame, for instance in the roles of service user and service provider (Fox, 2018). These types of divisions tend to disregard mutual relationships of non-family members based on sharing and care (Fox, 2018). Furthermore, bureaucratic organisations like CCGs perceive these types of care as riskier than more traditionally delivered services (Fox, 2018). Fox (2018) argues that health and social care provision in the UK is akin to placing our most vulnerable in invisible asylums: they are excluded from sharing power and resources, and from having any meaningful autonomy. Instead Fox (2018), argues that the value of care services is produced through relationships between people. Service users and providers together create spaces and experiences that promote health and wellbeing.

Therapeutic nursing homes

The nursing home sector has attempted to overcome negative stereotypes, including associations with decline, degeneration and frailty, with neglect (Braedley, 2018), as well as – particularly since COVID-19 – with death. Previous efforts to redesign care homes to be akin to hotels or other familiar settings have unfortunately reconstructed the power dynamics of previous forms (Braedley, 2018). However, one UK nursing home for people with dementia did attempt to challenge such dynamics, creating a community where music, decoration and even food was delivered therapeutically (Braedley, 2018). Meaningful relationships were the most important part of the community, providing residents with dignity and a sense of self (Braedley, 2018). Residents and staff share spaces such as kitchens, preparing food and interacting with each other, while volunteers (family and friends) assist with activities like gardening (Braedley, 2018). This anti-institutional and de-professionalising model produces an 'equitable, respectful, inclusive alternative … that promote[d] communal, collective living that includes family, residents, workers and volunteers' (Braedley, 2018: 57). Following COVID-19, calls to radically rethink and reimagine the structure and ethos of residential homes have grown in momentum:

> The way forward must certainly be to 'downsize' from 'industrial scale' care, looking at placing the running and financing of homes (with 20 residents maximum) into the hands of residents, staff and family members: co-operative care in all but name. Tightly regulated foster

care, as a complementary strategy, may be another option. Crucially, such homes should develop strong (preferably intergenerational) links with groups in the surrounding community. (Phillipson, 2020b)

Following a broadcast on Channel Four in 2017 called *Old People's Home for 4 Year Olds*, about a US intergenerational care scheme trialled in the UK, there has been recent interest in residential settings for older people that have intergenerational elements of care. Filmed over six weeks, the programme captured the physical, emotional and social wellbeing of both the four-year-olds and the residents (The ExtraCare Charitable Trust, 2018). The intergenerational friendships fostered during the series, while doing a number of shared activities, were reported to have had a positive effect on the health and wellbeing of the residents (The ExtraCare Charitable Trust, 2018). There is evidence that intergenerational contact with non-family members can improve the cognitive ability of older people (Dury et al, 2017). It is exactly these types of innovative schemes, in a safe post-COVID-19 context, that would be worth developing and exploring.

Age-friendly cities: alternative public health

Although initiatives relating to age-friendly cities and communities have existed since the 1990s, it was only in 2010 that the WHO provided guidance on what being age-friendly actually means, as notions of 'ageing in place' started to emerge within the health and social care sector (Thomese et al, 2018). At this time, Manchester created an age-friendly cities and communities (AFCC) programme and the Old Moat project came to fruition (White and Hammond, 2018). The aims of the project were simple: to find out what was and was not age-friendly about the Old Moat area, and then to work with the local community to make it more so (White and Hammond, 2018). The project's methodology was designed to fully involve older residents in decision-making about the social and physical design (White and Hammond, 2018). The genuine involvement of the residents in designing an urban space resulted in the development of age-friendly neighbourhoods (White and Hammond, 2018). Such socially and politically active participation of people in later life is the original holistic aim of the WHO's framework for active ageing ('the process of optimising opportunities for health, participation and security in order to enhance the quality of life as people age' [WHO, 2002: 12]), rather than the narrow focus on physical functioning promoted by many health professionals (see Chapters 2 and 5). Furthermore, with ageing populations becoming more diverse (particularly in urban settings), and as the power structures of racism and ageism intersect, greater numbers of older people from minority ethnic communities will become isolated and precarious (Buffel et al, 2018). Therefore, age-friendly cities, communities and design could be key to addressing discrimination based on age, gender, ethnicity and class (Buffel et al, 2018). These new ways of imagining urban spaces for the benefit of older residents do, however, rely on investment from local authorities, whose budgets have been under significant pressure both before and during the pandemic (Ogden et al, 2020).

Relational/asset-based approaches

A final example of innovatively reimagining health and social care are relational and asset-based approaches. One such approach is called Human, Learning, Systems (HLS) (Lowe et al, 2020). This has been described as an 'alternative paradigm for funding, commissioning and management of human service interventions in complex systems' (Lowe et al, 2020: 251). It is a response to the complexity that exists in the health and social care system, and is underpinned by a relational, human-centred approach to understanding the strengths and needs of people (Lowe et al, 2020). It aims to understand people's heterogenicity, build empathy, build on people's assets (rather than defects) and trust professionals to act altruistically (Lowe et al, 2020). It suggests that learning rather than services be commissioned, and the aims to build trusting relationships, find common ground and acknowledge the role that commissioners play as gatekeepers of the commissioning system (Low et al, 2020). This kind of approach has been trialled in a nursing home in the Netherlands, where nurses self-managed themselves to assess the strengths and needs of the residents, and to respond in a bespoke manner (Laloux, 2014). The performance of the nurses is peer-reviewed to enhance the service (Laloux, 2014). Relational approaches to care services are at their heart reciprocal rather than transactional, and lead to revolutionary ways of thinking about the way spaces and interactions are harnessed in care settings (Cottam, 2020). Since COVID-19, there has been a stronger call for a cultural shift from deficit- to asset-based approaches to care, whereby communities are conceptualised as a collective of active citizens rather than passive recipients (Russell, 2020).

Key issues of cultural change

Quality, holistic and reciprocal relationships

Firstly, what these examples of innovation have in common is a focus on the quality of relationships between people, whether they are related or not. This is why outcomes-based approaches are far superior, as they focus on what care means subjectively to particular individuals. Whether it is making someone a cup of tea, listening to someone talk about their day or a simple hug, what care means to people is socially and culturally constructed, and that is what process-based models do not capture.

Secondly, the relationships engendered by these models are holistic, as they do not reduce older people to their physical or biological functions. Instead, the whole person is considered, including their psychological and social wellbeing (Burns et al, 2016b).

Thirdly, the interactions are reciprocal: the older person is not reduced to a passive entity 'to' whom something is done. Instead, they are treated as someone 'with' whom something is done (Barnes et al, 2018). There is an exchange of activity, interaction, knowledge, experience or feeling that demonstrates the agency of both parties (Sevenhuijsen, 1998). There are several ways in which these changes can be made to how older people experience health and social care, from intergenerational living, therapeutic care homes, age-friendly cities and relational/asset-based commissioning, but moving on from the tragedy of COVID-19, there is a unique opportunity for transformation and change. It has highlighted our interdependence and collective responsibility, like never before; 'COVID-19 and lockdown have taken us to a moment of viscerally experiencing our interdependence: in shared risk, shared care, shared experience' (Melville and Wilkinson, 2020: 40). This interdependency is something that populations in the UK are culturally resistant to. Perhaps changing these attitudes could be the legacy of the COVID-19 pandemic.

Care ethics and precarious interdependence

As Barnes et al (2018: 28) write, 'we have a collective responsibility for individuals in need because we all need care at some times in our lives'. Care is relational and interdependent, but also political (Sevenhuijsen, 1998) – the ways in which people are cared for, and care for others, are shaped by global discourse, national policy and regional implementation. For instance, as stated previously, older people can care about their social and physical environment and be part of the decision-making to develop age-friendly cities, but only when in the presence of political discourse, policies and the will to enable them. Furthermore, Grenier (2020), drawing on Butler (2009), argues that vulnerability is an inevitable part of one's life; physical limitations can affect someone throughout the lifecourse, whether as a result of ageing, illness, disease or disability. Therefore, this book argues that three cultural changes are necessary in order to shift the political discourses around health and social care for older people.

Firstly, care for people in later life must be seen as a collective responsibility of society, and the organisation of that care must change from the neoliberal, individualistic and negligent processes currently carried out by low-paid and poorly resourced staff. Secondly, precariousness and vulnerability are not fixed end-states applied to older people, but universal human experiences. This understanding should be embedded into health and social care policy, to enhance empathy and understanding between groups or individuals. Finally, health and social care for older people should be understood in the context of precarious interdependence rather than in terms of dependency relationships. Cultures in the Global North must shift their thinking from ageist tropes of dependency and frailty in later life towards understanding that both precarity and dependence are part of the human condition, and not just applicable to older people. Reconceptualising older people's care in these ways opens up possibilities for political action and social solidarity (Fine, 2020). Unlike the health and social care crisis, the COVID-19 pandemic is universal; it has touched everyone in some way and opened people's eyes to the failings of the health and social care system. This new public understanding needs to be harnessed to ensure a radical reconfiguration of care in later life.

A Moonshot feminist approach to health and social care

Mazzucato (2021) argues that to fix 'wicked' problems, such as health and social care, governments must be reimagined and reconfigured to achieve the mission. This should begin with the restructuring of welfare states around the principle of universal care for all, while resisting and reversing the unjust neoliberal marketisation of care systems (The Care Collective, 2020). Waves of feminism have highlighted the injustices of care work being feminised, devalued and not recognised as 'work' (Hayes, 2017). Yet, women are still providing most of the care for relatives in the family, as well as in outside agencies, being paid to provide care services in either domiciliary settings or within residential institutions (Bunting, 2020). Thus, the historical connotations of care work being of low value and feminised have continued (Hayes, 2017). Care systems need to be opened up to new collective ways of thinking, which move away from outdated notions of care as 'women's work' to broader conceptualisations of providing care within interdependent communities (The Care Collective, 2020). Much like some of the innovative alternative health and social care models discussed previously, missions are about risk-taking via innovation and learning (Mazzucato, 2021). Our Moonshot mission, as I see it, is to use the momentum from the COVID-19 pandemic and the ways in which health and social care work has been *re*-valued, to reconceptualise 'care' as interdependent, indispensable and life-sustaining, particularly in later life.

Appendices

Appendix 1: Methodology for Case Study 1

Case Study 1 has been extracted from the author's doctoral thesis (Simmonds, 2011). It utilised a narrative inquiry to capture older people's experiences about physical activity in a rural area of the UK. The research started in June 2007 and was completed in November 2011. Seven focus groups, 20 in-depth interviews, 16 activity diaries (capturing physical activity experiences), and 19 re-interviews with visual elicitation (using healthy living leaflets, see Appendix 3 for an example) were triangulated. Data was analysed inductively using thematic analysis. For a more detailed account of the methodology, see Simmonds (2011).

Appendix 2: Research team and methodology for Case Study 2

Methodology for paramedic participant data

This qualitative study was nested within a feasibility trial exploring whether paramedics could administer a questionnaire about fracture risk to patients who had fallen (ISRCTN36245726). The fieldwork was based in an English Ambulance Foundation Trust and data collection took place between August 2013 and February 2014 (for the protocol, see Clarke et al, 2014). The qualitative study comprised methods observing practice by shadowing paramedics, followed by semi-structured interviews. Bethany Simmonds [BS] (Research Fellow) signed confidentiality statements and governance assurances were in place. Potential participants of both genders and with a range of years of experience were purposely sampled using the list of paramedics involved in the feasibility trial; they were sent study information packs and then telephoned about participation. Paramedics indicated whether they were interested in taking part and those who were completed consent forms. In total, 14 paramedics were approached and all agreed to take part. Data collection ceased when saturation was reached and no new themes emerged.

In eight sessions of shadowing, BS observed paramedics' everyday practice. Eight of these paramedics were interviewed during or after the shadowing and a further six paramedics were interviewed at another time. Paramedics were observed while they attended patients over 50 years who had fallen. Observation was chosen as a useful method because of the situation, interplay between different organisations, and emotional reactions of both the paramedics and patients to the situation and how it unfolded. BS took observational field notes, including details about delivering the intervention, discussion of treatment options, advice or education provided about self-care, and how paramedics coordinated with other service providers. The field notes were subsequently typed up and anonymised.

In 14 interviews, BS asked paramedics about their experience and training, experience of participating in the study (including recruitment of patients and delivering the intervention) and their reflections on the important aspects of care for older people who fall. A flexible topic guide allowed for inductive data to emerge from participants. With written informed consent (including for publication of anonymised quotations), audio recordings were made of the interviews. These were subsequently transcribed and anonymised. The interview transcripts and fieldwork notes were thematically coded, analysed separately and then together, with the aid of NVivo qualitative analysis software (version 10).

Methodology for patient participant data

This qualitative study took place within a feasibility trial exploring whether paramedics could administer a questionnaire about fracture risk to patients who had fallen (ISRCTN36245726). The fieldwork was based in an English Ambulance Foundation Trust and data collection took place between August 2013 and February 2014 (for the protocol, see Clarke et al, 2014).

Twenty semi-structured interviews with men and women over 50 years who had fallen and been attended to by a study paramedic were completed. Due to this research taking place in an emergency care setting where patients have fallen, sometimes lying on the floor for hours, called 999 and been attended to by a paramedic, we implemented a two-stage consent process for the trial. In the first stage of consent, paramedics first met the patients' clinical needs, helped them to become comfortable and then asked eligible patients or a personal consultee (carer or family member) if they were interested in taking part in some research preventing people from falling and breaking their bones. If the patient or a personal consultee acting on their behalf agreed, they completed the FRAX questionnaire and gave permission for BS to contact them at a later date to give them more information about the trial. Patients who were admitted to hospital for 24 hours or more following the fall became ineligible and their formal consent was not sought. In the second stage of consent, BS contacted eligible patients or their personal consultees to discuss the research. Potential participants were sent packs with further information about the study, and if they wanted to participate, they provided their consent at a later date in writing by post or in a face-to-face meeting.

Patients confirmed whether they were still interested in taking part in an interview by returning the reply slip and or the consent form. All participants provided written consent to the interview at the time of the interview itself or had returned the consent form with the reply slip. In total, 33 patients were sent information packs about the qualitative interview study. Interviews took place an average of 15 weeks after participants had given their verbal agreement to their participation in the trial.

Fourteen semi-structured interviews were undertaken with patients deemed to have the capacity to consent to research, and six with family members or care staff for patients (personal consultees) who were identified by paramedics as lacking mental capacity to consent. In 20 interviews, BS asked patients or their consultee about their or the patient's fall when they or the patient was attended by the ambulance; if the patient had fallen previously or subsequently; whether they remembered being asked the FRAX questions, and if so, how they experienced this; whether they remembered being asked for verbal consent to be in the trial, if so, how they experienced this; how they felt about being asked to see their GP (if in intervention arm); how they felt about randomisation and subsequent differential care; how did they find completing study the questionnaires; and finally why they decided to take part in the study. Visual elicitation was also used to prompt participants' memory of completing the study materials. This is where visual material, such as a copy of the questionnaire, is used to provide stimulus for discussion in the interview (Simmonds, 2011). A flexible topic guide allowed for inductive data to emerge from participants. With written informed consent (including publication of anonymised quotations), audio recordings were made of the interviews. They were subsequently transcribed and anonymised. Data collection ceased when saturation was reached, and no new themes emerged. The interview transcripts were analysed thematically with the aid of NVivo qualitative analysis software (version 10).

Research team

The OAK Project team consisted of the following members: Dr Bethany Simmonds, Dr Shane Clarke (principal investigator), Dr Rachel Bradley, Ms Maria Robinson, Professor Rachael Gooberman-Hill, Ms Sarah Black, Professor Christopher Salisbury, Professor Jonathan Benger, Dr Elsa Marques, Professor Lee Shepstone, Mrs Rosemary Greenwood, Dr Elinor Griffiths and Ms Sandra Mulligan. All the authors acknowledge and are grateful for the support of the English Ambulance Service Trust that facilitated this research, as well as the Research Design Service and University Hospitals Bristol NHS Foundation Trust for their support in carrying out this study. The OAK Project team would also like to acknowledge the support of the National Institute for Health Research, through the Comprehensive Clinical Research Network.

Ethics approval

This study was given a favourable opinion by the NRES Committee South Central – Oxford C. REC reference: 12/SC/0604 on the 31st of October 2012.

Funding

This article presents independent research funded by the National Institute for Health Research (NIHR) under its Research for Patient Benefit (RfPB) Programme (Grant Reference Number PB-PG-0711-25070). The views expressed are those of the author(s) and not necessarily those of the NHS, the NIHR or the Department of Health.

Appendix 3: Example of a healthy ageing leaflet: Chichester District Council (no date) *HeartSmart Walks: Walk for your Hearts sake*, Chichester District Council: Chichester

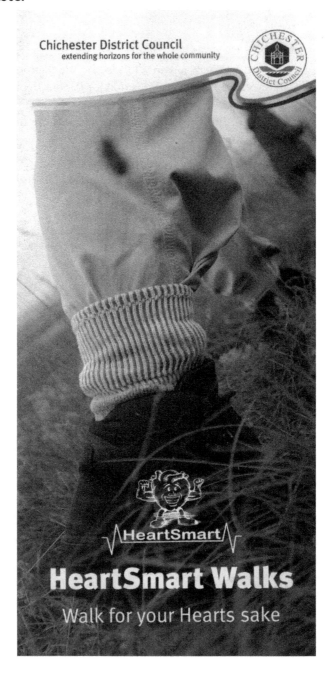

References

AACE [Association of Ambulance Chief Executives] (2011) 'Taking Healthcare to the Patient 2: A review of six years progress and recommendations for the future', Available from: http://aace.org.uk/wp-content/uploads/2015/05/taking_healthcare_to_the_patient_2.pdf

Adkins, L. and Holland, J. (eds) (1996) *Sex, Sensibility and the Gendered Body*, London: Macmillan.

Agamben, G. (2005) *State of Exception*, London: Palgrave.

Age UK (2020) 'Behind the headlines: time to bring our care workers in from the cold', Available from: https://www.ageuk.org.uk/globalassets/age-uk/documents/reports-and-publications/time-to-bring-our-care-workers-in-from-the-cold-2nd-november-2020.pdf

AIUK [Amnesty International UK] (2020) 'As if expendable: the UK government's failure to protect older people in care homes during the COVID-19 pandemic', Available from: https://www.amnesty.org.uk/files/2020-10/Care%20Homes%20Report.pdf

AIUK [Amnesty International UK] (2021) 'CQC report does not go far enough on DNR scandal', Available from: https://www.amnesty.org.uk/press-releases/uk-cqc-report-does-not-go-far-enough-dnr-scandal

Albert, A. (2019) 'Matt Hancock says social care green paper will stop people moving to care homes unless "clinically justified"', *homecare.co.uk*, 1 May, Available from: https://www.homecare.co.uk/news/article.cfm/id/1609244/Matt-Hancock-says-social-care-green-paper-will-stop-people-entering-care-homes

Alcock, P. (2010) 'The Big Society: a new policy environment for the third sector?', in C. Pierson, F. Castles and U. Naumann (eds) *The Welfare State Reader* (3rd edn), Oxford: Wiley, pp 296–308.

Anderson, B. (2010) 'Migration, immigration controls and the fashioning of precarious workers', *Work, Employment and Society*, 24(2): 300–17.

Anderson, C. (2020) '"You're shirking responsibility!" BBC host rages at work from home advice at minister', *Express*, 17 July, Available from: https://www.express.co.uk/news/uk/1310692/bbc-james-brokenshire-work-from-home-advice-latest-update

Andersson, G. and Karlberg, I. (2000) 'Integrated care for the elderly: the background and effects of the reform of Swedish care of the elderly', *International Journal of Integrated Care*, 1(1): 1–10.

Anttonen, A. and Karsio, O. (2017) 'How marketisation is changing the Nordic model of care for older people', in F. Martinelli, A. Anttonen and M. Matzke (eds) *Social Services Disrupted: Changes, Challenges and Policy Implications for Europe in Times of Austerity*, Cheltenham: Edward Elgar Publishing, pp 219–38.

Arber, S. and Ginn, J. (1994) 'Women and aging', *Reviews in Clinical Gerontology*, 4(4): 349–58.

Arber, S. and Ginn, J. (1998) 'Health and illness in later life', in D. Field and S. Taylor (eds) *Sociological Perspectives on Health, Illness and Health Care*, Oxford: Blackwell Science Ltd pp 134–51.

Aronsson, K., Bjorkdahl, I. and Wireklint, B. (2013) 'Prehospital emergency care for patients with suspected hip fractures after falling – older patients' experiences', *Journal of Clinical Nursing*, 23(21–22): 3115–23.

Association of Directors of Adult Services (2014) 'ADASS budget survey report 2014: final', Available from: https://www.thinklocalactpersonal. org.uk/_assets/News/July/ADASS_Budget_Survey_Report_2014_ Final.pdf

Asthana, A. and Elgot, J. (2017) 'Theresa May ditches manifesto plan with "dementia tax" U-turn', *The Guardian*, 22 May, Available from: https:// www.theguardian.com/society/2017/may/22/theresa-may-u-turn-on-dementia-tax-cap-social-care-conservative-manifesto

Atkinson, C. and Crozier, S. (2020) 'Fragmented time and domiciliary care quality', *Employee Relations: The International Journal*, 42(1): 35–51.

Atkinson, C. and Lucas, R. (2013) 'Worker responses to HR practice in adult social care in England', *Human Resource Management Journal*, 23(3): 296–312.

Ayalon, Y. and Tesch-Romer, C. (2018) (eds) *Contemporary Perspectives on Ageism*, New York: Springer Open.

Bahle, T. (2003) 'The changing institutionalization of social services in England and Wales, France and Germany: is the welfare state on the retreat?', *Journal of European Social Policy*, 13(1): 5–20.

Ballanger, C. and Payne, C. (2002) 'The construction of the risk of falling among and by older people', *Ageing and Society*, 22(3): 305–24.

Baltes, P.B. and Mayer, K.U. (1999) *The Berlin Aging Study: Aging from 70 to 100*, New York: Cambridge University Press.

Bambra, C. (ed) (2019) *Health in Hard Times: Austerity and Health Inequalities*, Bristol: Policy Press.

Barnes, M., Gahagan, B. and Ward, L. (2018) *Re-imagining Old Age: Wellbeing, Care and Participation*, Malaga, Spain: Vernon Press.

Barr, C., Davis, N. and Duncan, P. (2021) 'UK coronavirus deaths pass 100,000 after 1,564 reported in one day', *The Guardian*, 13 January, Available at: https://www.theguardian.com/world/2021/jan/13/ uk-coronavirus-deaths-pass-100000

Barron, D. and West, E. (2017) 'The quasi-market for adult residential care in the UK: do for-profit, not-for-profit or public sector residential care and nursing homes provide better quality care?', *Social Science and Medicine*, 179: 137–46.

Bauman, Z. (1998) *Globalization: The Human Consequences*, Cambridge: Polity Press.

Bazalgette, L. and Salter, J. (2013) 'Sociable housing in later life', *Homeshare*, Available from: http://homeshare.org/wp-content/uploads/2012/04/Sociable-Housing-in-Later-Life-May13.pdf

BBC (2020) 'Coronavirus: above-inflation pay rise for almost 900,000 public sector workers', *BBC News*, 21 July, Available from: https://www.bbc.co.uk/news/business-53478404

Beck, U. (1999) *What is Globalization?* Cambridge: Polity Press.

Beech, M. and Lee, S. (eds) (2015) *The Conservative-Liberal Coalition: Examining the Cameron-Clegg Government*, Basingstoke: Palgrave Macmillan.

Bell, D., Comas-Herrera, A., Henderson, D., Jones, S., Lemmon, E., Moro, M., Murphy, S., O'Reilly, D. and Patrignani, P. (2020) 'COVID-19 mortality and long-term care: a UK comparison', *CPEC-LSE*, 29 August, Available from: https://ltccovid.org/wp-content/uploads/2020/08/COVID-19-mortality-in-long-term-care-final-Sat-29-1.pdf

Beveridge, W. (1942) 'Social Insurance and Allied Services' (Beveridge Report), London: HMSO.

Bisley, N. (2007) *Rethinking Globalization*, Basingstoke: Palgrave Macmillan.

BMA [British Medical Association] (2020) 'COVID-19: the risk to BAME doctors', *British Medical Association*, 18 June. Available from: https://www.bma.org.uk/advice-and-support/covid-19/your-health/covid-19-the-risk-to-bame-doctors

Bochel, H. and Powell, M. (2016) *The Coalition Government and Social Policy*, Bristol: Policy Press.

Bottery, S., Ward, D. and Fenny, D. (2019) 'Social Care 360', London: The Kings Fund. Available at: https://www.kingsfund.org.uk/sites/default/files/2019-05/social-care-360-pdf.pdf?utm_source=website&utm_medium=social&utm_term=thekingsfund&utm_content=pdfreport&utm_campaign=socialcare360

Bourdieu, P. (1977) *Outline of a Theory of Practice*, Cambridge: Cambridge University Press.

Bourdieu, P. (1984) *Distinction: A Social Critique of the Judgement of Taste*, London: Routledge.

Bourdieu, P. (1986) 'The forms of capital', in J. E. Richardson (ed) *Handbook of Theory for Research in the Sociology of Education*, Westport, CT: Greenwood Press, pp 241–58.

Bourdieu, P. (1987) 'What makes a social class? On the theoretical and practical existence of groups', *The Berkeley Journal of Sociology*, 32: 1–18.

Bourdieu, P. (1998) *Acts of Resistance: Against the Tyranny of the Market*, New York: The New Press and Policy Press.

Bowman, A., Erturk, I., Folkman, P., Fround, J. Haslam, C., Johal, S., Leaver, A., Moran, M., Tsitsianis, N. and Williams, K. (2015) *What a Waste: Outsourcing and How It Goes Wrong*, Manchester: Manchester University Press.

Braedley, S. (2018) 'Reinventing the nursing home: metaphors that design care', in S. Katz (ed) *Ageing in Everyday Life: Materialities and Embodiments*, Bristol: Bristol University Press, pp 45–61.

Brennan, D., Cass, B., Himmelweit, S., and Szebehely, M. (2012) 'The marketization of care: rationales and consequences in Nordic and liberal care regimes', *Journal of European Social Policy*, 22(4): 377–91.

Brimblecombe, P. (1987) *The Big Smoke: A History of Air Pollution in London since Medieval Times*, London: Methuen.

Brown, J.M. (2015) 'Northamptonshire council takes outsourcing to different level', *The Financial Times*, 12 April. Available from: https://www.ft.com/content/c642439c-dfa1-11e4-a6c4-00144feab7de

BSG [British Society for Gerontology] (2020) 'BSG Statement on COVID-19: 20 March 2020'. Available from: https://www.britishgerontology.org/publications/bsg-statements-on-covid-19/statement-one

Buffel, T., Doran, P., Lewis, C., Phillipson, C. and Yarker, S. (2020) 'Covid-19: bringing the social back in', *Ageing Issues*, 16 April. Available from: https://ageingissues.wordpress.com/2020/04/16/covid-19-bringing-the-social-back-in/

Buffel, T., Handler, S. and Phillipson, C. (2018) 'Age-friendly cities and communities: a manifesto for change', in T. Buffel, S. Handler and C. Phillipson (eds) *Age-Friendly Cities and Communities: A Global Perspective*, Bristol: Policy Press, pp 273–88.

Bulmer, C. (2010) 'Homeshare research report', Cumbria: Homeshare Steering Group Committee.

Bunting, M. (2020) *Labours of Love: Crisis in Care*, London: Granta.

Burns, D., Cowie, L., Earle, J., Folkman, P., Froud, J., Hyde, P., Johal, S., Rees Jones, I., Killett, A. and Williams, K. (2016a) 'Where does the money go? Finalised chains and the crisis in residential care', Manchester and Milton Keynes: Centre for Research on Socio-Cultural Change. Available from: http://hummedia.manchester.ac.uk/institutes/cresc/research/WDTMG%20FINAL%20-01-3-2016.pdf

Burns, D., Earle, J., Folkman, P., Froud, J., Hyde, P., Johal, S., Rees Jones, I., Killett, A. and Williams, K. (2016b) 'Why we need social innovation in home care for older people', Manchester and Milton Keynes: Centre for Research on Socio-Cultural Change. Available from: http://hummedia.manchester.ac.uk/institutes/cresc/research/social-innovation-in-home-care.pdf

Burrows, R., Nettleton, S. and Bunton, R. (2005) 'Health, risk and consumption under late modernism', in R. Bunton, S. Nettleton and R. Burrows (eds) *The Sociology of Health Promotion: Critical Analyses of Consumption, Health and Risk*, London: Routledge, pp 1–8.

Bury, M. (1991) 'The sociology of chronic illness: a review of research and prospects', *Sociology of Health and Illness*, 13(4): 451–68.

Buser, B., Amelung V.E. and Schneider, N. (2008) 'German community pastors' contact with palliative care patients and collaboration with health care professionals', *Journal of Social Work in End-Of-Life & Palliative Care*, 4(2): 85–100.

Busse, R. and Riesberg, A. (2004) 'Health care systems in transition: Germany', Copenhagen: WHO Regional Office for Europe on behalf of the European Observatory on Health Systems and Policies.

Butler, E. and Saper, P. (2020) 'Fixing social care: new funding, new methods, new partnerships', London: Adam Smith Institute. Available from: https://www.adamsmith.org/s/Fixing-social-care-Eamonn-Butler-and-Paul-Saper-Final.pdf

Butler, J. (2004) *Precarious Life: The Powers of Mourning and Violence*, London: Verso.

Butler, J. (2009) *Frames of War: When is a Life Grievable?*, London: Verso.

Cabinet Office (2020) 'Guidance: making a Christmas bubble with friends and family', gov.uk, 31 December. Available from: https://www.gov.uk/government/publications/making-a-christmas-bubble-with-friends-and-family/making-a-christmas-bubble-with-friends-and-family

Cabinet Office (2021) 'Guidance: national lockdown: stay at home', gov.uk, 28 January. Available from: https://www.gov.uk/guidance/national-lockdown-stay-at-home#summary-what-you-can-and-cannot-do-during-the-national-lockdown

Cahill, D. and Konings, M. (2017) *Neoliberalism: Key Concepts*, Cambridge: Polity Press.

Calasanti, T. (2007) 'Bodacious berry, potency wood and the aging monster: Gender and age-relations in anti-ageing ads', *Social Forces*, 86(1): 335–55.

Calasanti, T. (2015) 'Combating ageism: how successful is successful aging?', *The Gerontologist*, 56(6): 1093–101.

Calasanti, T. (2020a) 'Brown slime, the silver tsunami, and apocalyptic demography: the importance of ageism and age relations', *Social Currents*, 7(3): 195–211.

Calasanti, T. (2020b) 'Pervasive ageism in the response to the pandemic (aging and the life course), *Footnotes*, 48(3). Available from: https://www.asanet.org/news-events/footnotes/may-jun-2020/research-policy/pervasive-ageism-response-pandemic-aging-and-life-course

Calvert, J. and Arbuthnott, G. (2021) *Failures of State: The Inside Story of Britain's Battle with Coronavirus*, London: Harper Collins Publishers.

Camerer, C.F. and Hogarth, R. (1999) 'The effects of financial incentives in experiments: a review and capital-labor-production framework', *Journal of Risk and Uncertainty*, 19(1): 7–42.

Campbell, D. (2020) 'Boris Johnson plans radical shake-up of NHS in bid to regain more direct control', *The Guardian*, 10 July. Available from: https://www.theguardian.com/society/2020/jul/10/boris-johnson-plans-radical-shake-up-of-nhs-in-bid-to-regain-more-direct-control

Campbell, I. and Price, R. (2016) 'Precarious work and precarious workers: towards an improved conceptualisation', *The Economic and Labour Relations Review*, 27(3): 314–32.

Carers UK (2020a) 'Research: the forgotten families in lockdown: unpaid carers close to burnout during Covid-19 crisis', Press release, *Carers UK*, 23 April. Available from: https://www.carersuk.org/news-and-campaigns/press-releases/research-the-forgotten-families-in-lockdown-unpaid-carers-close-to-burnout-during-covid-19-crisis

Carers UK (2020b) 'Caring behind closed doors: six months on: the continued impact of the coronavirus (COVID-19) pandemic on unpaid carers', *Carers UK*, October 2020. Available from: http://www.carersuk.org/images/News_and_campaigns/Behind_Closed_Doors_2020/Caring_behind_closed_doors_Oct20.pdf

Carney, G.M. and Nash, P. (2020) *Critical Questions for Ageing Societies*, Bristol: Policy Press.

Carroll, W.D., Strenger, V., Eber, E., Porcaro, F., Cutrera, R., Fitzgerald, D.A. and Balfour-Lynn, I.M. (2020) 'European and United Kingdom COVID-19 pandemic experience: the same but different', *Paediatric Respiratory Reviews*, 35: 50–6. Available from: https://doi.org/10.1016/j.prrv.2020.06.012

Carstein, B. (2003) 'Economic evaluation of Homeshare', Victoria, Australia: Homeshare.

Centre for Ageing Better (2020) 'An old age problem? How society shapes and reinforces negative attitudes to ageing', 3 November. Available from: https://www.ageing-better.org.uk/news/uks-damaging-views-ageing-revealed-new-report-analysing-language-used-across-society

Chappell, N.L. and Havens, B. (1980) 'Old and female: testing the double jeopardy hypothesis', *The Sociology Quarterly*, 21(2): 157–71.

Charles, A. (2020) 'Integrated care systems explained: making sense of systems, places and neighbourhoods', *The King's Fund*, 8 April. Available from: https://www.kingsfund.org.uk/publications/integrated-care-systems-explained

Charles, A. and Ewbank, L. (2020) 'The road to renewal: five priorities for health and care', *The King's Fund*, 16 July. Available from: https://www.kingsfund.org.uk/publications/covid-19-road-renewal-health-and-care

Chilton, M.A. (2004) 'Brief analysis of trends in prehospital care services and a vision for the future', *Australian Journal of Paramedicine*, 2(1): 1–7.

Clarke, J. (2008) 'Living with/in and without neo-liberalism', *Focall-European Journal of Anthropology*, 51: 135–47.

Clarke, S., Bradley, R., Simmonds, B., Salisbury, C., Benger, J., Marques, E., Greenwood, R., Shepstone L., Robinson, M., Appleby-Fleming, J., and Gooberman-Hill, R. (2014) 'Can ambulance paramedics use FRAX® (the WHO Fracture Risk Assessment Tool) to help GPs improve future fracture risk in patients that fall?', *BMJ Open*, 4(9): 1–9.

Clasen, J. and Gould, A. (1995) 'Stability and change in welfare states: Germany and Sweden in the 1990s', *Policy and Politics*, 23(3): 189–202.

Clements, L. (2017) 'The Care Act overview', 11 January. Available from: https://www.readingmencap.org.uk/media/1138/care-act-notes-updated-jan2017.pdf

Coffey, J. (2010) 'An evaluation of Homeshare pilot programmes in West Sussex, Oxfordshire and Wiltshire', Oxford: Oxford Brookes University. Available from: https://radar.brookes.ac.uk/radar/file/f1de7010-faf5-1783-b9bb-a3fb5ff44dea/1/coffey2010evaluation.pdf

College of Paramedics (2015) 'Scope of practice', Bristol: College of Paramedics. Available from: https://collegeofparamedics.co.uk/COP/ProfessionalDevelopment/Scope_of_Practice.aspx

Comas-Herrera, A., Zalakaín, J., Litwin, C., Hsu, A.T., Lemmon, E., Henderson, D. and Fernández, J-L. (2020) 'Mortality associated with COVID-19 outbreaks in care homes: early international evidence', London: International Long-Term Care Policy Network, CPEC-LSE. Available from: https://ltccovid.org/wp-content/uploads/2020/06/Mortality-associated-with-COVID-among-people-who-use-long-term-care-26-June.pdf

Corus, C. and Saatcioglu, B. (2015) 'An intersectionality framework for transformative services research', *The Service Industries Journal*, 35(7–8): 415–29.

Cottam, H. (2020) 'Welfare 5.0: why we need a social revolution and how to make it happen', London: Institute for Innovation and Public Purpose. Available at: https://www.ucl.ac.uk/bartlett/public-purpose/sites/public-purpose/files/iipp_welfare-state-5.0-report_hilary-cottam_wp-2020-10_final.pdf

Coupland, V.H., Madden, P., Jack, R.H., Mollerm H. and Davies, E.A. (2011) 'Does place of death from cancer vary between ethnic groups in South East England?', *Palliative Medicine*, 25(4): 314–22.

CQC [Care Quality Commission] (2010) 'The state of health care and adult social care in England: key themes and quality of services in 2009', London: The Stationery Office.

CQC [Care Quality Commission] (2017) 'State of care: the state of health care and adult social care in England 2017/18', Available at: https://webarchive.nationalarchives.gov.uk/20190112070317/https://www.cqc.org.uk/publications/major-report/state-care

CQC [Care Quality Commission] (2019) 'Adult inpatient survey 2019'. Available at: https://www.cqc.org.uk/publications/surveys/adult-inpatient-survey-2019

CQC [Care Quality Commission] (2020) 'Review of Do Not Attempt Cardiopulmonary Resuscitation decisions during the Covid-19 pandemic: interim report', November. Available at: https://www.cqc.org.uk/publications/themed-work/review-do-not-attempt-cardiopulmonary-resuscitation-decisions-during-covid

CQC [Care Quality Commission] (2021) 'Protect, respect, connect – decisions about living and dying well during COVID-19: CQC's review of "do not attempt cardiopulmonary resuscitation" decisions during the COVID-19 pandemic', final report, March. Available at: https://www.cqc.org.uk/publications/themed-work/protect-respect-connect-decisions-about-living-dying-well-during-covid-19

Crawford, R. (1980) 'Healthism and the medicalization of everyday life', *International Journal of Health Services*, 10(3): 365–88.

Crawford, R. Stoye, G. and Zaranko, B. (2020) 'What impact did cuts to social care spending have on hospitals?', *Institute for Fiscal Studies*, 7 December. Available at: https://www.ifs.org.uk/publications/15214#:~:text=We%20find%20that%20cuts%20to,over%20the%20eight%2Dyear%20period

Crenshaw, K. (1989) 'Demarginalizing the intersection of race and sex: a black feminist critique of antidiscrimination doctrine, feminist theory and antiracist politics', *University of Chicago Legal Forum*, 1(8): 139–68.

Cumming, E. and Henry, W.E. (1961) *Growing Old*, New York: Basic.

Darzi, A. (2018) 'Better health and care for all: a 10-point plan for the 2020s', London: Institute for Public Policy Research. Available from: https://www.ippr.org/research/publications/better-health-and-care-for-all

Davidsson, J.B. (2018) 'Dualising the Swedish model: insiders and outsiders and labour market policy reform in Sweden: an overview', in S. Theodoropoulou (ed) *Labour Market Reforms in the Era of Pervasive Austerity: A European Perspective*, Bristol: Policy Press, pp 169–95.

Davies, W. (2017) *The Limits of Neoliberalism: Authority, Sovereignty and the Logic of Competition*, London: SAGE.

Davis, N. (2020) 'Kamikaze': the experts urging UK to rethink Christmas Covid rules', *The Guardian*, 15 December. Available from: https://www.theguardian.com/politics/2020/dec/15/kamikaze-the-experts-urging-uk-to-rethink-christmas-covid-rules

Dayan, M. (2017) 'Getting a Brexit deal that works for the NHS', *The Nuffield Trust*, 31 May. Available from: https://www.nuffieldtrust.org.uk/files/2017-05/getting-brexit-deal-for-nhs-web-final.pdf

de Best, R. (2021) 'Coronavirus (COVID-19) deaths worldwide per one million population as of January 29, 2021, by country', *Statista*, 29 January. Available from: https://www.statista.com/statistics/1104709/coronavirus-deaths-worldwide-per-million-inhabitants/

Dean, M. (2010) *Governmentality: Power and Rule in Modern Society*, London: SAGE.

Dean, M. (2013) *The Signature of Power: Sovereignty, Governmentality and Biopolitics*, London: SAGE.

Department of Health Statistical Service (1999) 'Statistical bulletin: ambulance services, England: 1998–9', Bulletin 1999/16, London: Department of Health.

DH [Department of Health] (1989a) 'Caring for people: community care in the next decade and beyond', London: HMSO.

DH [Department of Health] (1989b) 'Working for patients', London: HMSO.

DH [Department of Health] (1991) 'The patients' charter', London: HMSO.

DH [Department of Health] (1997) 'The new NHS: modern, dependable', London: Stationary Office.

DH [Department of Health] (1998) 'Modernising social services: promoting independence, improving protection, raising standards', London: Stationery Office.

DH [Department of Health] (2004) 'At least five times a week: evidence on the impact of physical activity and its relationship to health', London: Department of Health. Available from: https://webarchive.nationalarchives.gov.uk/20130105001829/http://www.dh.gov.uk/prod_consum_dh/groups/dh_digitalassets/@dh/@en/documents/digitalasset/dh_4080981.pdf

DH [Department of Health] (2008a) 'End of life care strategy: promoting high quality care for all adults at the end of life', London: Department of Health. Available from: https://www.gov.uk/government/uploads/system/uploads/attachment_data/file/136431/End_of_life_strategy.pdf

DH [Department of Health] (2008b) 'High quality care for all: NHS next stage review final report', London: TSO.

DH [Department of Health] (2011) 'Factsheet 5: physical activity guidelines for older adults (65+ years)', London: Department of Health. Available from: https://www.gov.uk/government/uploads/system/uploads/attachment_data/file/213741/dh_128146.pdf

DH [Department of Health] (2019) 'UK chief medical officers' physical activity guidelines', London: Department of Health. Available from: https://assets.publishing.service.gov.uk/government/uploads/system/uploads/attachment_data/file/832868/uk-chief-medical-officers-physical-activity-guidelines.pdf

DHSC [Department of Health and Social Care] (2018) 'The adult social care workforce in England', London: National Audit Office. Available from: https://www.nao.org.uk/wp-content/uploads/2018/02/The-adult-social-care-workforce-in-England.pdf

DHSC [Department of Health and Social Care] (2020) 'Guidance: coronavirus (COVID-19): care home support package', gov.uk, 15 May. Available from: https://www.gov.uk/government/publications/coronavirus-covid-19-support-for-care-homes

DHSC [Department of Health and Social Care] (2021a) 'Transforming the public health system: reforming the public health system for the challenges of our times', policy paper, 29 March. Available from: https://www.gov.uk/government/publications/transforming-the-public-health-system/transforming-the-public-health-system-reforming-the-public-health-system-for-the-challenges-of-our-times?utm_source=The%20King%27s%20Fund%20newsletters%20%28main%20account%29&utm_medium=email&utm_campaign=12258293_NEWSL_HWB_2021-04-05&dm_i=21A8,7AQK5,VPIPLS,TLLBH,1

DHSC [Department of Health and Social Care] (2021b) 'Integration and innovation: working together to improve health and social care for all', policy paper, 11 February. Available from: https://www.gov.uk/government/publications/working-together-to-improve-health-and-social-care-for-all/integration-and-innovation-working-together-to-improve-health-and-social-care-for-all-html-version

Dickinson, A., Horton, K., Machen, I., Bunn, F., Cove, J., Jain, D., Maddex, T. et al (2011) 'The role of health professionals in promoting the uptake of fall prevention interventions: Aa qualitative study of older people', *Age and Ageing*, 40(6): 724–30.

Dixton, S. Smith, C. and Touchet, A. (2018) 'The disability perception gap: policy report', SCOPE, May. Available from: http://www.scope.org.uk/scope/media/files/campaigns/disability-perception-gap-report.pdf

Dorling, D. (2014) 'Why are the old dying before their time? How austerity has affected mortality rates', *New Statesman*, 13 February. Available from: https://www.newstatesman.com/politics/2014/02/why-are-old-people-britain-dying-their-time

Douglas, C. (1992) 'For all the saints', *BMJ*, 304: 579.

Dowding, K. (2020) 'Is Johnson's government bailing out from responsibility?', *Transforming Society*, 14 May. Available from: http://www.transformingsociety.co.uk/2020/05/14/is-johnsons-government-bailing-out-from-responsibility/

Dumas, A. and Laberge, S. (2005) 'Social class and ageing bodies: understanding physical activity in later life', *Social Theory & Health*, 3: 183–205.

Dumas, A. and Turner, B.S. (2006) 'Age and ageing: The social world of Foucault and Bourdieu', in J. Powell and A. Wahidin (eds) *Foucault and Aging*, Hauppauge, NY: Nova Science Publishers, pp 145–56.

Dury, L., Abrams, D and Swift, H.J. (2017) 'Making intergenerational connections – an evidence review: what are they, why do they matter and how to make more of them', Age UK. Available from: https://www.ageuk. org.uk/globalassets/age-uk/documents/reports-and-publications/reports-and-briefings/active-communities/rb_2017_making_intergenerational_ connections.pdf

Eichhorst, W. and Hassel, A (2018) 'Are there austerity-related policy changes in Germany?', in S. Theodoropoulou (ed) *Labour Market Reforms in the Era of Pervasive Austerity: A European Perspective*, Bristol: Policy Press, pp 115–68.

Elli Finance (UK) Plc and Elli Investments Limited (2021) 'ANNOUNCEMENT'. Available from: https://www.fshc.co.uk/media/ 23258/announcement-21-june-2021-call-details.pdf

Erlandsson, S., Storm, P., Stranz, A., Szebehely, M. and Trydeggard, G. (2013) 'Marketising trends in Swedish eldercare: competition, choice and calls for stricter regulation', in G. Meagher and M. Szebehely (eds) *Marketization in Nordic Eldercare: A Research Report on Legislation, Oversight, Extent and Consequences*, Stockholm: Stockholm University Press, pp 23–84.

Esping-Andersen, G. (1990) *The Three Worlds of Welfare Capitalism*, Princeton, NJ: Princeton University Press.

Estes, C. (1979) *The Aging Enterprise*, San Francisco: Jossey Bass.

Estes, C.L. and Binney, E. A (1989) 'The biomedicalization of aging: dangers and dilemmas', *The Gerontologist*, 29(5): 587–96.

Estes, C.L. and Wallace, S.P. (2010) 'Globalization, social policy and ageing: a North American perspective', in D. Dannefer and C. Phillipson (eds) *The SAGE Handbook of Social Gerontology*, London: SAGE, pp 513–24.

Fast, J. and de Long Gierveld, J. (2008) 'Ageing, disability and participation', in N. Keating (ed) *Rural Ageing: A Good Place to Grow Old?*, Bristol: Policy Press, pp 63–75.

Ferguson, I. (2007) 'Increasing user choice or privatizing risk? The antinomies of personalization', *British Journal of Social Work*, 37: 387–403.

Fetzer, T. (2020) 'Subsidizing the spread of COVID19: evidence from the UK's Eat-Out-to-Help-Out scheme', CAGE working paper no. 517, October. Available at: https://warwick.ac.uk/fac/soc/economics/research/ centres/cage/manage/publications/wp.517.2020.pdf

Fine, M. (2020) 'Reconstructing dependency: precarity, precariousness and care in old age', in A. Grenier, C. Phillipson and R.A. Settersten (eds) *Precarity and Ageing: Understanding Insecurity and Risk in Later Life*, Bristol: Policy Press, pp 169–89.

Fisher, L. (2018) 'Winter 2017/18: the worst ever for the NHS?', *Full Fact*, 23 May. Available from: https://fullfact.org/health/winter-201718-worst-ever-nhs/

Foucault, M. (1972) *The Archaeology of Knowledge*, London: Tavistock Publications.

Foucault, M. (1978) *The History of Sexuality, Volume 1: An Introduction*, London: Penguin Books.

Foucault, M. (1991) *Discipline and Punish*, London: Penguin Books.

Foucault, M. (2008) *The Birth of Biopolitics: Lectures at the College De France, 1978–79*, M. Senellart (ed), Basingstoke: Palgrave Macmillan.

Fox, A. (2018) *A New Health and Care System: Escaping the Invisible Asylum*, Bristol: Policy Press.

France, A. (2020) 'Germany in coronavirus lockdown again with schools closed and drinking in public banned', *Evening Standard*, 13 December. Available from: https://www.standard.co.uk/news/world/germany-lockdown-again-coronavirus-b287842.html

Gardner, T. and Fraser, C. (2021) 'Longer waits, missing patients and catching up: how is elective care in England coping with the continuing impact of COVID-19?', *The Health Foundation*, 13 April. Available from: https://www.health.org.uk/news-and-comment/charts-and-infographics/how-is-elective-care-coping-with-the-continuing-impact-of-covid-19?utm_source=The%20King%27s%20Fund%20newsletters%20%28main%20account%29&utm_medium=email&utm_campaign=12297356_NEWSL_HMP%202021-04-13&dm_i=21A8,7BKP8,VPIPLS,TQ47E,1

Gilleard, C. (2018) 'Suffering: the darker side of ageing', *Journal of Aging Studies*, 44: 28–33.

Gilleard, C. (2020) 'Bourdieu's forms of capital and the stratification of later life', *Journal of Aging Studies*, 53: 100851.

Gilleard, C. and Higgs, P. (2011) 'Ageing abjection and embodiment in the fourth age', *Journal of Aging Studies*, 25(2): 135–42.

Givati, A. Markham, C. and Street, K. (2018) 'The bargaining of professionalism in emergency care practice: NHS paramedics and higher education', *Advance in Health Science Education*, 23: 353–69.

Glasby, J. (2003) *Hospital Discharge: Integrating Health and Social Care*, Abington: Radcliffe Medical Press.

Glasby, J. (2017) *Understanding Health and Social Care*, Bristol: Policy Press.

Glasby, J. (2019) *The Short Guide to Health and Social Care*, Bristol: Policy Press.

GMB (2011) 'Southern Cross: the cross we have to bear, the greedy and the gullible', London: GMB.

GMB (2020) 'Poor PPE to blame for thousands of ambulance workers Covid-19 absences', 19 November. Available from: https://www.gmb.org.uk/printpdf/2161

Godlee, F. (2016) 'How Jeremy Hunt derailed clinician led progress towards a seven day NHS', *BMJ*, 352: 1–4.

Goodley, S. (2011) 'Southern Cross care fiasco sheds light on secretive world of private equity', *The Guardian*, 3 June. Available from: https://www.theguardian.com/business/2011/jun/03/southern-cross-care-private-equity

Graham, H. (2009) *Understanding Health Inequalities* (2nd edn), Maidenhead: Open University Press.

Grant, B.C. (2002) 'Deliberate physical activity as a form of leisure in the later years second draft', unpublished paper, Hamilton, New Zealand: Waikato University.

Green, M., Dorling, D., and Minton, J. (2017) 'The geography of a rapid rise in elderly mortality in England and Wales, 2014–15', *Heath and Place*, 44: 77–85.

Grenier, A., Lloyd, L. and Phillipson, C. (2017a) 'Precarity in late life: rethinking dementia as a "frailed" old age', *Sociology of Health and Illness*, 39(2): 318–30.

Grenier, A., Phillipson, C., Rudman, D.L., Hatzifilalithis, S., Kobayashi, K. and Marier, P. (2017b) 'Precarity in late life: understanding new forms of risk and insecurity', *Journal of Aging Studies*, 43: 9–14.

Grenier, A. (2020) 'Rereading frailty through a lens of precarity: an explication of politics and the human condition of vulnerability', in A. Grenier, C. Phillipson and R.A. Settersten (eds) *Precarity and Ageing: Understanding Insecurity and Risk in Later Life*, Bristol: Policy Press, pp 69–90.

Grenier, A., Phillipson, C. and Settersten, R.A. (2020a) 'Precarity and ageing: new perspectives for social gerontology', in A. Grenier, C. Phillipson and R.A. Settersten (eds) *Precarity and Ageing: Understanding Insecurity and Risk in Later Life*, Bristol: Policy Press, pp 1–15.

Grenier, A., Phillipson, C. and Settersten, R.A. (eds) (2020b) *Precarity and Ageing: Understanding Insecurity and Risk in Later Life*, Bristol: Policy Press.

Griffiths, R. (1988) *Community Care: Agenda for Action* (Griffiths Report), London: HMSO.

Grohls, S., Schneiders, K. and Heinze, R.G. (2015) 'Social entrepreneurship versus intrapreneurship in the German social welfare state: a study of old-age care and youth welfare services', *Nonprofit and Voluntary Sector Quarterly*, 44(1): 163–80.

Ham, C. and Charles, A. (2018) 'Accountable care is a promising way of integrating care', *The BMJ Opinion*, 30 January. Available from: https://blogs.bmj.com/bmj/2018/01/30/chris-ham-and-anna-charles-accountable-care-is-a-promising-way-of-integrating-care/

Hamad, H. (2020) 'NHS workers and the UK media in the time of Covid-19', *Soundings Blog*, 20 April. Available from: https://www.lwbooks.co.uk/soundings/blog/nhs-workers-and-the-uk- media-in-the-time-of-covid-19

Hanlon, N. and Poulin, L. (2021) 'Rural health and ageing: making way for a critical gerontology of rural health', in M. Skinner, R. Winterton and K. Walsh (eds) *Rural Gerontology: Toward Critical Perspectives on Rural Ageing*, London: Routledge, pp 40–51.

Hardin, C. (2014) 'Finding the "neo" in neoliberalism', *Cultural Studies*, 28(2): 199–221.

Harding, R., Epiphaniou, E. and Chidgey-Clark, J. (2012) 'Needs, experience and preferences of sexual minorities for end-of-life care and palliative care: a systematic review', *Palliative Medicine*, 15(5): 602–11.

Harrington, C., Jacobsen, F.F., Panos, J., Pollock, A., Sutaria, S. and Szebehely, M. (2017) 'Marketization in long-term care: a cross-country comparison of large for-profit nursing home chains', *Health Services Insights*, 10:1–23.

Harrison, S and McDonald, R. (2008) *The Politics of Healthcare in Britain*, London: SAGE.

Harrop, E., Farnell, D., Longo, M., Goss, S., Sutton, E., Seddon, K., Nelson, A., Byrne, A. and Selman, L. (2020) 'Supporting people bereaved during COVID-19: study report 1', Cardiff University and the University of Bristol, 27 November. Available from: https://www.covidbereavement.com/

Harvey, D. (2005) *A Brief History of Neoliberalism*, Oxford: Oxford University Press.

Hassel, A. and Schiller, C. (2010) *Der Fall Hartz IV: Wie es zur Agenda 2010 kam und wie es weitergeht*, Frankfurt/Main: Campus Verlag.

Havighurst, R. (1961) 'Successful aging', *The Gerontologist*, 1(1): 8–13.

Hayes, L.J.B. (2017) *Stories of Care: A Labour of Law*, London: Palgrave.

Health Policy Insight (2021) 'Editorial Friday 5 February 2021: exclusive – government's new health white paper draft text', *Health Policy Insight*, 5 February. Available from: http://www.healthpolicyinsight.com/?q=node/1699

Healthwatch and British Red Cross (2020) '590 people's stories of leaving hospital during COVID-19', *Healthwatch*, 20 October. Available from: https://www.healthwatch.co.uk/report/2020-10-27/590-peoples-stories-leaving-hospital-during-covid-19

Hepworth, M. (1995) 'Positive ageing: what is the message?', in R. Bunton, S. Nettleton and R. Burrows (eds) *The Sociology of Health Promotion*, London: Routledge, pp 176–90

Hiam, L., Harrison, D., McKee, M. and Dorling, D. (2018) 'Why is life expectancy in England and Wales "stalling"?', *Journal of Epidemiology and Community Health*, 72(5): 404–8.

Higgs, P. and Gilleard, C. (2014) 'Frailty, abjection and the "othering" of the fourth age', *Health Sociology Review*, 23(1): 10–19.

Higgs, P. and Gilleard, C. (2015) *Re-thinking Old Age: Theorising the Fourth Age*, London: Palgrave.

HM Treasury (2019) 'Almost a million public sector workers handed a second year of inflation-busting pay rises', gov.uk, 22 June. Available from: https://www.gov.uk/government/news/almost-a-million-public-sector-workers-handed-a-second-year-of-inflation-busting-pay-rises

Hodgson, K., Grimm, F., Vestesson, E., Brine, R. and Deeny, S. (2020) 'Adult social care and COVID-19: assessing the impact on social care users and staff in England so far', The Health Foundation. Available from: https://www.health.org.uk/sites/default/files/upload/publications/2020/20200730-Adult-social-care-and-COVID-19-impact-so-far.pdf

Hokema, A. (2017) 'Extended working lives in Germany from a gender and life-course perspective: a country in policy transition', in A.I. Leime, D. Street, S. Vickerstaff, C. Krekula and W. Loretto (eds) *Gender, Ageing and Extended Working Life: Cross-National Perspectives*, Bristol: Policy Press, pp 99–116.

Holmes, J. (2021) 'Brexit and the end of the transition period: what does it mean for the health and care system?', *The King's Fund*, 11 January. Available from: https://www.kingsfund.org.uk/publications/articles/brexit-end-of-transition-period-impact-health-care-system#trade

Holstein, M. (2011) 'Cultural ideals, ethics and agelessness: a critical perspective on the third age', in D. Carr and K. Komp (eds) *Gerontology in the Era of the Third Age: Implications and Next Steps*, New York: Springer Publishing, pp 225–44.

Horton, A. (2019) 'Financialization and non-disposable women: real estate, debt and labour in UK care homes', *EPA: Economy and Space*, July: 1–16, Available from: doi: 10.1177/0308518X19862580.

Horton, R. (2020) *The Covid-19 Catastrophe: What's Gone Wrong and How to Stop It Happening Again*, Cambridge: Polity Press.

House of Commons (2020) 'Social care: funding and workforce: third report of session 2019–21', House of Commons Health and Social Care Committee, 13 October. Available at: https://committees.parliament.uk/publications/3120/documents/29193/default/

Howarth, G. (2007) *Death and Dying: A Sociological Introduction*, Cambridge: Polity Press.

Hudson, B. (2014) 'Dealing with market failure: a new dilemma in UK health and social care policy?', *Critical Social Policy*, 35(2): 281–92.

Hudson, B. (2019) 'Commissioning for change: a new model for commissioning adult social care in England', *Critical Social Policy*, 39(3): 413–33.

Hughes, J., Chester, H. and Challis, D. (2009) 'Recruitment and retention of a social care workforce for older people', Personal Social Services Research Unit, Discussion Paper M193–2.

Humphries, R., Thorlby, R., Holder, H., Hall, P. and Charles, A. (2016) 'Social care for older people: some home truths', London: The King's Fund. Available from: https://www.kingsfund.org.uk/publications/social-care-older-people

Hunter, D.J. (2008) *The Health Debate* (2nd edn), Bristol: Policy Press.

Hurd Clarke, L. (2010) *Facing Age*, Lanham, MD: Rowham and Littlefield.

Hyde, M. and Higgs, P. (2017) *Ageing and Globalisation*, Bristol: Policy Press.

Jack, S. (2017) 'The crisis: 10 years in three charts', BBC News, 9 August, Available from: www.bbc.co.uk/news/business-40869369

Jacobi, L. and Kluve, J. (2007) 'Before and after the Hartz reforms: the performance of active labour market policy in Germany', *Journal for Labour Market Research*, 40(1): 45–64.

James, L. (2020) 'Circuit-breaker lockdown: what is it and what would it look like?', *The Independent*, 7 October. Available from: https://www.independent.co.uk/news/uk/home-news/circuit-breaker-lockdown-coronavirus-uk-scotland-b500116.html

Jarman, H. and Greer, S.L. (2015). 'The big band: health and social care reform under the coalition', in M. Beech and S. Lee (eds) *The Conservative-Liberal Coalition: Examining the Cameron-Clegg Government*, Basingstoke: Palgrave Macmillan, pp 50–68.

Jimenez-Beatty Navarro, J.E., Graupera Sanz, J.L., del Castillo, J.M., Izquierdo, A.C. and Rodriguez, M.M. (2007) 'Motivation factors and physician advice for physical activity in older urban adults', *Journal of Aging and Physical Activity*, 15(3): 241–56.

Jox, R.J., Krebs, M., Fegg, M., Reiter-Theil, S., Frey, L., Eisenmenger, W. and Borasio, G.D. (2010) 'Limiting life-sustaining treatment in German intensive care units: a multiprofessional survey', *Journal of Critical Care*, 25(3): 413–19.

Karlsson, C-J. (2020) 'Sweden's coronavirus failure started long before the pandemic', *Foreign Policy*, 23 June. Available from: https://foreignpolicy.com/2020/06/23/sweden-coronavirus-failure-anders-tegnell-started-long-before-the-pandemic/

Katz, S. (1996) *Disciplining Old Age: The Formation of Gerontological Knowledge*, Charlottesville: University of Virginia Press.

Katz, S. (2000) 'Busy bodies: activity, aging and the management of everyday life', *Journal of Aging Studies*, 14(2): 135–52.

Katz, S. (2005) *Cultural Aging: Life Course, Lifestyle and Senior Worlds*, Peterborough, ON: Worldview Press.

Katz, S. (2018) (ed) *Ageing in Everyday Life: Materialities and Embodiments*, Bristol: Policy Press.

Katz, S. and Calasanti, T. (2015) 'Critical perspectives on successful aging: does it "appeal more than it illuminates"?', *The Gerontologist*, 55(1): 26–33.

Kessler, D., Peters, T.J., Lee, L. and Parr, S. (2005) 'Social class and access to specialist palliative care services', *Palliative Medicine*, 19(2): 105–10.

Kirby, T. (2020) 'Evidence mounts on the disproportionate effect of COVID-19 on ethnic minorities', *The Lancet/Respiratory Medicine*. Available from: DOI:https://doi.org/10.1016/S2213-2600(20)30228-9

Kotecha, V. (2019) Plugging the leaks in the UK care home industry: strategies for resolving the financial crisis in the residential and nursing home sector', Centre for Health and the Public Interest. Available from: https://chpi.org.uk/wp-content/uploads/2019/11/CHPI-PluggingTheLeaks-Nov19-FINAL.pdf

Krekula, C., Engstrom, L-G. and Alvinius, A. (2017) 'Sweden: an extended working life policy that overlooks gender considerations', in A.I. Leime, D. Street, S. Vickerstaff, C. Krekula and W. Loretto (eds) *Gender, Ageing and Extended Working Life: Cross-National Perspectives*, Bristol: Policy Press, pp 157–74.

Krekula, C. and Johansson, B. (eds) (2016) 'Inledning' [Introduction], in C. Krekula and B. Johansson (eds) *Introduktion till kritiska åldersstudier* [Introduction to Critical Age Studies], Malmö, Sweden: Studentlitteratur.

Krekula, C., Nikander, P. and Wilińska, M. (2018) 'Multiple marginalizations based on age: gendered ageism and beyond', in L. Ayalon and C. Tesch-Römer (eds) *Contemporary Perspectives on Ageing*, New York: Springer Open, pp 33–50.

Laberge, S. and Kay, K. (2002) 'Pierre Bourdieu's sociocultural theory and sport practice', in J. Maguire and K. Young (eds) *Theory, Sport and Society*, London: Elsevier, pp 239–66.

Lain, D. (2018) *Reconstructing Retirement: Work and Welfare in the UK and USA*, Bristol: Polity Press.

Lain, D., Airey, L., Loretto, W. and Vickerstaff, S. (2020) 'Older workers and ontological precarity: between precarious employment, precarious welfare and precarious households', in A. Grenier, C. Phillipson and R.A. Settersten (eds) *Precarity and Ageing: Understanding Insecurity and Risk in Later Life*, Bristol: Policy Press, pp 91–114.

Laloux, F. (2014) *Reinventing Organizations: A Guide to Creating Organizations Inspired by the Next Stage in Human Consciousness*, Brussels: Nelson Parker.

Lamb, S. (2014) 'Permanent personhood or meaningful decline? Toward a critical anthropology of successful aging', *Journal of Aging Studies*, 29: 41–52.

Laslett, P. (1989) *A Fresh Map of Life: The Emergence of the Third Age*, Cambridge, MA: First Harvard University Press.

Lassen, A.J. and Moreira, T. (2014) 'Unmaking old age: political and cognitive formats of active ageing', *Journal of Aging Studies*, 30: 33–46.

Laugaland K., Aase, K. and Barach, P. (2012) 'Interventions to improve patient safety in transitional care – a review of the evidence', *Work*, 41(1): 2915–24.

Lawrence, D. (2020) 'An avoidable crisis: the disproportionate impact of Covid-19 on Black, Asian and minority ethnic communities', The Labour Party. Available from: https://www.lawrencereview.co.uk/

Le Grand, J. (2007) *The Other Invisible Hand: Delivering Public Services Through Choice and Competition*, Princeton, NJ and Oxford: Princeton University Press.

Lee, S. (2011) '"We are all in this together": the coalition agenda for British modernization', in S. Lee and M. Beech (eds) *The Cameron-Clegg Government: Coalition Politics in an Age of Austerity*, Basingstoke: Palgrave Macmillan, pp 3–24.

Lee, S. (2015) 'Indebted and unbalanced: the political economy of the Coalition', in M. Beech and S. Lee (eds) *The Conservative-Liberal Coalition: Examining the Cameron-Clegg Government*, Basingstoke: Palgrave Macmillan, pp 16–36.

Leitner, S. (2003) 'Varieties of familialism: the caring function of the family in comparative perspective', *European Societies*, 5(4): 353–75.

Levi, S., Wurm, S. and Ayalon, Y. (2018) 'Origins of Ageism at the Individual Level', in Y. Ayalon and C. Tesch-Romer (eds) *Contemporary Perspectives on Ageism*, New York: Springer Open, pp 51–72.

Liang, J. and Luo, B. (2012) 'Toward a discourse shift in social gerontology: from successful aging to harmonious aging', *Journal of Aging Studies*, 26(3): 327–34.

Lowe, T., French, M. and Hawkins, M. (2020) 'The human, learning, systems approach to commissioning in complexity', in A. Bonner (ed) *Local Authorities and the Social Determinants of Health*, Bristol: Policy Press, pp 241–62.

Lund, B. (2007) 'The state' in M. Powell (ed) *Understanding the Mixed Economy of Welfare* (2nd edn), Bristol: Policy Press, pp 41–63.

Lupton, D. (1995) *The Imperative of Health: Public Health and the Regulated Body*, London: SAGE.

Macmillan, R. and Rees, J. (2007) 'Voluntary and community welfare', in M. Powell (ed) *Understanding the Mixed Economy of Welfare* (2nd edn), Bristol: Policy Press, pp 91–112.

Macnicol, J. (2015) *Neoliberalising Old Age*, Cambridge: Cambridge University Press.

McIntyre, N., Batty, D. and Duncan, P. (2020) 'Fears grow student Covid infections will spread into local areas in England and Wales', *The Guardian*, 12 October. Available from: https://www.theguardian.com/education/2020/oct/12/fears-grow-student-covid-infections-england-wales-will-spread-into-local-communities

McCann, L., Granter, E., Hyde, P. and Hassard, J. (2013) 'Still blue-collar after all these years? An ethnography of the professionalization of emergency ambulance work', *Journal of Management Studies*, 50(5): 750–76.

McKenna, H. (2021) 'The health and social care White Paper explained', The Kings Fund. Available from: https://www.kingsfund.org.uk/publications/health-social-care-white-paper-explained?utm_source=The%20King%27s%20Fund%20newsletters%20%28main%20account%29&utm_medium=email&utm_campaign=12235808_NEWSL_The%20Weekly%20Update%202021-03-12&utm_content=white_paper_explainer&dm_i=21A8,7A97K,VPIPLS,TJGW5,1

Mahase, E. (2020) 'Covid-19: what have we learnt about the new variant in the UK?', *BMJ*, 371: m4944. Available from: https://doi.org/10.1136/bmj.m4944

Markula, P. (2003) 'The technologies of the self: sport, feminism and Foucault', *Sociology of Sport*, 20(2): 87–107.

Marmot, M., Allen, J., Goldblatt, P., Herd, E. and Morrison, J. (2020) *Build Back Fairer: The COVID-19 Marmot Review. The Pandemic, Socioeconomic and Health Inequalities in England*, London: Institute of Health Equity.

Mason, R. (2020) 'Boris Johnson boasted of shaking hands on day Sage warned not to', *The Guardian*, 5 May. Available from: https://www.theguardian.com/politics/2020/may/05/boris-johnson-boasted-of-shaking-hands-on-day-sage-warned-not-to

Mazzucato, M. (2021) *Mission Economy: A Moonshot Guide to Changing Capitalism*, Rushton, UK: Penguin Random House.

Mbembe, A (2003) 'Necropolitics', *Public Culture*, 15(1): 11–40.

Mercille, J. (2017) 'Neoliberalism and health care: the case of the Irish nursing home sector', *Critical Public Health*, 28(5): 546–59.

Metro US (2021) 'Germany's vaccine rollout gets shot in the arm from doctors surgeries', *Metro US*, 8 April. Available from: https://www.metro.us/germanys-vaccine-rollout-gets/

Millar, K.L. (2017) 'Towards a critical politics of precarity', *Social Compass*, 11(6): e12483.

Miller, R. (2007) 'Market welfare', in M. Powell (ed) *Understanding the Mixed Economy of Welfare* (2nd edn), Bristol: Policy Press, pp 65–90.

Mirowski, P. (2013) *Never Let a Serious Crisis Go to Waste: How Neoliberalism Survived the Financial Meltdown*, London: Verso.

Mirowski, P. and Plehwe, D. (eds) (2009) *The Road from Mont Pèlerin: The Making of the Neoliberal Thought Collective*, Cambridge, MA: Harvard University Press.

Mishra, R. (1999) *Globalization and the Welfare State*, Cheltenham: Edward Elgar Publishing.

Moran, M. (1999) *Governing the Health Care State: A Comparative Study of the United Kingdom, the United States and Germany*, Manchester: Manchester University Press.

Murray, J. (2020) 'The five-day Christmas Covid bubble: how will it work?', *The Guardian*, 24 November. Available from: https://www.theguardian.com/world/2020/nov/24/the-five-day-christmas-covid-bubble-how-will-it-work

Murray, R. (2021) 'The King's Fund's response to plans for the future public health system in England', The King's Fund, 26 April. Available at: https://www.kingsfund.org.uk/publications/future-public-health-system-england

Murray, R., Edwards, N. and Dixon, J. (2019) 'The impact of a no deal Brexit on health and care: An open letter to MPs', The King's Fund, 3 September, Available from: https://www.kingsfund.org.uk/publications/no-deal-brexit

Myles, J. (1984) *Old Age in the Welfare State: The Political Economy of Public Pensions*, Lawrence: University Press of Kansas.

National Audit Office (2014) 'Adult social care in England: overview', 13 March, London: National Audit Office.

National Audit Office (2015) 'Sustainability and financial performance of acute hospital trusts', 16 December, London: National Audit Office.

National Audit Office (2018) 'The adult social care workforce in England', 8 February, London: National Audit Office.

National Audit Office (2021) 'The adult social care market in England', 25 March, London: Department of Health and Social Care. Available from: https://www.nao.org.uk/report/adult-social-care-markets/

National Health Service Confederation (2014) 'Ripping off the sticking plaster: whole-system solutions for urgent and emergency care', 6 March, London: NHS Confederation. Available from: https://www.nhsconfed.org/-/media/Confederation/Files/Publications/Documents/ripping-off-the-sticking-plaster.pdf

National Health Service Improvement (2019) 'Performance of the NHS provider sector for the year ended 31 March 2019'. Available from: https://improvement.nhs.uk/documents/5404/Performance_of_the_NHS_provider_sector_for_the_quarter_4_1819.pdf#page=33

Nettleton, S. and Bunton, R. (2005) 'Sociological critiques of health promotion', in R. Bunton, S. Nettleton and R. Burrows (eds) *The Sociology of Health Promotion: Critical Analyses of Consumption, Health and Risk* (2nd edn), London: Routledge, pp 35–54.

NHS England [National Health Service] (2017) 'Next steps on the NHS five year forward view', 31 March. Available from: https://www.england.nhs.uk/publication/next-steps-on-the-nhs-five-year-forward-view/

NHS England [National Health Service] (2019) 'The NHS long term plan', January. Available from: https://www.longtermplan.nhs.uk/wp-content/uploads/2019/08/nhs-long-term-plan-version-1.2.pdf

NHS England [National Health Service] (2021) 'COVID-19 vaccination statistics: week ending Sunday 1st August 2021'. Available from: https://www.england.nhs.uk/statistics/wp-content/uploads/sites/2/2021/08/COVID-19-weekly-announced-vaccinations-05-August-2021.pdf

NIHR [National Institute for Health Research] (2018) 'The proportion of patients not transported to emergency departments after an ambulance is called varies across the country', 2 October. Available from: https://discover.dc.nihr.ac.uk/content/signal-000652/nationally-around-half-of-people-making-urgent-calls-for-an-ambulance-are-not-taken-to-hospital

Norman, A. (1985) *Triple Jeopardy: Growing Old in a Second Home-land*, London: Centre for Policy on Ageing.

Ogden, K., Phillips, D. and Spiliotis J-C. (2020) 'COVID-19 and English council funding: what is the medium-term outlook?', The Institute for Fiscal Studies. Available at: https://www.ifs.org.uk/publications/15041

O'Meara, P. (2009) 'Paramedics marching towards professionalism', *Australian Journal of Paramedicine*, 7(1): 1–5.

Ong, A. (2006) *Neoliberalism as Exception: Mutations in Citizenship and Sovereignty*, Durham, NC: Duke University Press.

Orange, R. (2020) 'As Covid death toll soars ever higher, Sweden wonders who to blame', *The Guardian*, 20 December. Available from: https://www.theguardian.com/world/2020/dec/20/as-covid-death-toll-soars-ever-higher-sweden-wonders-who-to-blame

Parliamentary and Health Service Ombudsman (2016) 'A report of investigations into unsafe discharge from hospital', May. Available from: https://www.ombudsman.org.uk/publications/report-investigations-unsafe-discharge-hospital-0

Parviainen, J. (2001) 'Women developing fitness products on the global market: the Method Putkisto Case', in P. Markula and E. Kennedy (eds) *Women and Exercise: The Body, Health and Consumerism*, London: Routledge, pp 44–60.

Paton, C. (2014) 'At what cost? paying the price for the market in the NHS', 17 February, London: Centre for Health in the Public Interest.

Paulson, S. and Willig, C. (2008) 'Older women and everyday talk about the ageing body', *Journal of Health Psychology*, 13(1): 106–20.

Peart, L. (2018) 'Four Seasons and H/2 Capital agree rescue deal terms', *Care Home Professional*, 21 May. Available from: https://www.carehomeprofessional.com/four-seasons-h-2-capital-agree-rescue-deal-terms/

Peston, R. (2011) 'The financial lessons of Southern Cross', *BBC News*, 2 June. Available from: www.bbc.co.uk/ news/business-13630394

PHE [Public Health England] (2020) 'Disparities in the risk and outcomes of COVID-19', 2 June. Available from: https://www.gov.uk/government/publications/covid-19-review-of-disparities-in-risks-and-outcomes

Philibert, I and Barach P. (2012) 'The European HANDOVER Project: A multi-nation program to improve transitions at the primary care-inpatient interface', *BMJ Quality and Safety*, 21(1): 1–6.

Phillips, D. (2019) 'The outlook for councils' funding: is austerity over?', Institute for Fiscal Studies, 11 November. Available from: https://www.ifs.org.uk/publications/14558

Phillipson, C. (1998) *Reconstructing Old Age: New Agendas in Social Theory and Practice*, London: SAGE.

Phillipson, C. (2015) 'The political economy of longevity: developing new forms of solidarity for later life', *The Sociological Quarterly*, 56(24): 1–10.

Phillipson, C. (2020a) 'Austerity and precarity: individual and collective agency in later life', in A. Grenier, C. Phillipson and R.A. Settersten (eds) *Precarity and Ageing: Understanding Insecurity and Risk in Later Life*, Bristol: Policy Press, pp 215–35.

Phillipson, C. (2020b) 'Covid-19 and the crisis in residential and nursing home care', *Ageing Issues*, 8 April. Available from: https://ageingissues.wordpress.com/2020/04/08/covid-19-and-the-crisis-in-residential-and-nursing-home-care/

Pickard, S. (2009) 'Frail bodies: geriatric medicine and the constitution of the fourth age', *Sociology of Health and Illness*, 36(4): 549–63.

Pike, E. (2010) 'Growing old (dis)gracefully? the gender/aging/exercise nexus', in P. Markula and E. Kennedy (eds) *Women and Exercise: The Body, Health and Consumerism*, London: Routledge, pp 180–96.

Pilmer, G. (2019) 'Care home operator Four Seasons appoints administrators', *Financial Times*, 30 April. Available from: https://www.ft.com/content/3dde7c20-6a79-11e9-80c7-60ee53e6681d

Platt, L. and Warwick, R. (2020) 'Are some ethnic groups more vulnerable to COVID-19 than others?', Institute for Fiscal Studies, 1 May. Available at: https://www.ifs.org.uk/inequality/chapter/are-some-ethnic-groups-more-vulnerable-to-covid-19-than-others/

Player, S. and Pollock, A. (2001) 'Long-term care: from public responsibility to private good', *Critical Social Policy*, s21(2): 231–55.

Pollitt, C. and Bouckaert, G. (2011) *Public Management Reform: A Comparative Analysis – New Public Management, Governance, and the Neo-Weberian State*, Oxford: Oxford University Press.

Powell J.L., Biggs, S. and Wahidin A. (2006) 'Exploring Foucault and bio-medical gerontology in western modernity', in J.L. Powell and A. Wahidin (eds) *Foucault and Aging*, Hauppauge, NY: Nova Science Publishers, pp 5–16.

Powell, J.L. and Wahidin, A. (2006) (eds) 'Introduction', in J.L. Powell and A. Wahidin (eds) *Foucault and Aging*, Hauppauge, NY: Nova Science Publishers, pp vii–xiii.

Rainey, N. (1998) 'Old age', in K. Trew and J. Kremler (eds) *Gender and Psychology*, London: Arnold, pp 153–64.

Raleigh, V. (2019) 'What is happening to life expectancy in the UK?', The King's Fund, 22 October. Available from: https://www.kingsfund.org.uk/publications/whats-happening-life-expectancy-uk

Razaq, A., Harrison, D., Karunanithi, S., Barr, B., Asaria, M., Routen, A. and Khunti, K. (2020) 'BAME Covid-19 deaths – what do we know? rapid data & evidence review', Centre for Evidence-Based Medicine, 5 May. Available from: https://www.cebm.net/covid-19/bame-covid-19-deaths-what-do-we-know-rapid-data-evidence-review/

Redwood, S., Simmonds, B., Fox, F., Shaw, A., Neubauer, K., Purdy, S. and Baxter, H. (2020) 'Consequences of "conversations not had": insights from a qualitative pilot study into failures in communication affecting delays in discharging older people living with frailty from hospital', *Journal of Health Services Research & Policy*, 25(4): 213–19. Available from: https://doi.org/10.1177%2F1355819619898229

Reintjes, R. (2020) 'Lessons in contact tracing from Germany', *British Medical Journal*, 369: m2522. Available from: http://dx.doi.org/10.1136/bmj.m2522

Research Councils UK (2009) 'Ageing: lifelong health and wellbeing'. Available from: https://mrc.ukri.org/research/initiatives/lifelong-health-wellbeing/

Rhodes, M. (1988) 'Globalization, labour markets and welfare states: a future of "competitive corporatism"?', in M. Rhodes and Y. Meny (eds) *The Future of European Welfare: A New Social Contract?*, London: Macmillan.

Ritzer, G. (2018) *The McDonaldization of society* (9th edn), London: SAGE.

Robertson, H. and Travaglia J. (2020) 'The necropolitics of COVID-19: will the COVID-19 pandemic reshape national healthcare systems?', *LSE Impact Blog*, 18 May. Available from: https://blogs.lse.ac.uk/impactofsocialsciences/2020/05/18/the-necropolitics-of-covid-19-will-the-covid-19-pandemic-reshape-national-healthcare-systems/

Rowe, J. and Kahn, R. (1987) 'Human aging: usual and successful', *Science*, 237(4811): 143–9.

Rubery, J., Grimshaw, D. and Hebson, G. (2013) 'Exploring the limits to local authority social care commissioning: competing pressures, variable practices, and unresponsive providers', *Public Administration*, 91(2): 419–37.

Russell, C. (2020) 'From deficit-based to asset-based community driven responses to Covid-19 (part 2)', *Nurture Development Blog*, 30 April. Available from: https://www.nurturedevelopment.org/blog/from-deficit-based-to-asset-based-community-driven-responses-to-covid-19-part-2/

Schmidt, M. (1982) 'The role of parties in shaping macro-economic policies', in F. Castles (ed) *The Impact of Parties*, London: SAGE.

Schmitter, P. and Lembruch, G. (eds) (1979) *Trends Towards Corporatist Intermediation*, London: SAGE.

Schulze, I. and Jochem, S. (2006) 'Germany: beyond gridlock', in E.M. Immergut, K.M. Anderson and I. Schulze (eds) *The Handbook of West European Pension Politics*, Oxford: Oxford University Press, pp 660–712.

Scourfield, P. (2011) 'Caretelization revisited and the lessons of Southern Cross', *Critical Social Policy*, 32(1): 137–48.

Settersten, R.A. (2020) 'How life course dynamics matter for precarity in later life', in A. Grenier, C. Phillipson and R.A. Settersten (eds) *Precarity and Ageing: Understanding Insecurity and Risk in Later Life*, Bristol: Policy Press, pp 19–40.

Sevenhuijsen, S. (1998) *Citizenship and the Ethics of Care: Feminist Considerations on Justice, Morality and Politics*, London: Routledge.

Seymour, J.E., Gott, M., Bellamy, G., Clark, D. and Ahmedzais, S.H. (2004) 'Planning for the end of life: the views of older people about advance care statements', *Social Science and Medicine*, 59(1): 57–68.

Seymour, J., Witherspoon, R., Gott, M., Ross, H., Payne, S. and Owen, T. (2005) *End-of-Life Care: Promoting Comfort, Choice and Well-Being for Older People*, Bristol: Policy Press.

Shalev, M. (1983) 'The social democratic model and beyond: two generations of comparative research on the welfare state', *Comparative Social Research*, 5: 315–51.

SharedLivesPlus (2016) 'Homeshare sector report: summer 2016'. Available from: https://homeshare.org/wp-content/uploads/Homeshare-Sector-Report-2016.pdf

Shilling, C. (2003) *The Body and Social Theory* (2nd edn), London: SAGE.

Simmonds, B.A.J. (2011) 'Experiences of physical activity in later life: making sense of embodiment, negotiating practicalities, and the construction of identities in rural spaces', PhD thesis, University of Southampton.

Sinclair, L. (2021) 'Germany coronavirus death toll tops 50,000 despite decrease in infections', *Evening Standard*, 22 January. Available from: https://www.msn.com/en-gb/news/newslondon/germany-coronavirus-death-toll-tops-50000-despite-decrease-in-infections/ar-BB1cZW3j

Skills for Care (2017) 'The state of the adult social care sector and workforce in England'. Available from: www.skillsforcare.org.uk

Smith, A. (1961 [1776]) *The Wealth of Nations*, E. Cannan (ed), London: Methuen.

Standing, G. (2011) *The Precariat: The Dangerous New Class*, London: Bloomsbury Academic.

Steger, M.B. and Roy, R.B. (2010) *Neoliberalism: A Very Short Introduction*, Oxford: Oxford University Press.

Stevenson, A. (2020) 'Shining a light on care homes during the COVID 19 pandemic in the UK 2020', *Quality in Ageing and Older Adults*, 21(4): 217–28.

Stewart, H., Sample, I. and Davis, N. (2021) 'New UK Covid variant may be 30% more deadly, says Boris Johnson', *The Guardian*, 23 January. Available from: https://www.theguardian.com/world/2021/jan/22/new-uk-covid-variant-may-be-more-deadly-says-boris-johnson

Stolt, R., Blomqvist, P. and Winblad, U. (2011) 'Privatization of social services: quality differences in Swedish elderly care', *Social Science and Medicine*, 72: 560–7.

Sudnow, D. (1967) *Passing On: The Social Organization of Dying*, Upper Saddle River, NJ: Prentice Hall.

Sundstrom, G. and Tortosa, M.A. (1999) 'The effects of rationing home-help services in Spain and Sweden: a comparative analysis', *Ageing and Society*, 19 (3): 343–61.

Swedish Pensions Agency (2016) 'Medelpensioneringsålder och utträdesålder' [Expected effective retirement age and retirement age], Stockholm: Fritzes.

The Care Collective (2020) *The Care Manifesto: The Politics of Independence*, London: Verso.

The ExtraCare Charitable Trust (2018) 'About the Show'. Available from: https://extracare.org.uk/channel-4-home-for/about-the-show/?

The Guardian (2020) 'Swedish PM says officials misjudged power of Covid resurgence', 15 December. Available from: https://www.theguardian.com/world/2020/dec/15/swedish-pm-says-officials-misjudged-power-of-covid-resurgence

The King's Fund (2020) 'The NHS budget and how it has changed', 13 March. Available from: https://www.kingsfund.org.uk/projects/nhs-in-a-nutshell/nhs-budget

The Local (2021) 'Covid infection rate in Germany goes up – but vaccines having impact on hospitalisations', 2 August. Available from: https://www.thelocal.de/20210802/covid-infection-rate-in-germany-goes-up-but-vaccines-having-impact-on-hospitalisations/

The Patients Association (2020) 'Premature discharge from hospital'. Available from: https://www.patients-association.org.uk/Handlers/Download.ashx?IDMF=e6cd54a0-5580-446d-ae98-9f6f7e8195b1

Thomas, C. (2007) *Sociologies of Disability and Illness: Contested Ideas in Disability Studies and Medical Sociology*, Basingstoke: Palgrave Macmillan.

Thomese, F., Buffel, T. and Phillipson, C. (2018) 'Neighbourhood change, social inequalities and age-friendly communities', in T. Buffel, S. Handler and C. Phillipson (eds) *Age-Friendly Cities and Communities: A Global Perspective*, Bristol: Policy Press, pp 33–49.

Thorlby, R., Starling, A., Broadbent, C. and Watt, T. (2018) 'What's the problem with social care, and why do we need to do better?', The Health Foundation, the Institute for Fiscal Studies, The King's Fund and the Nuffield Trust. Available from: https://www.health.org.uk/publications/nhs-at-70-what%E2%80%99s-the-problem-with-social-care-and-why-do-we-need-to-do-better

Thornton, J.E. (2002) 'Myths of ageing or ageist stereotypes', *Educational Gerontology*, 28(4): 301–12.

Timmins, N. (2012) 'Never again? the story of the Health and Social Care Act 2012: a study in coalition government and policy making', London: The Institute for Government and The King's Fund.

Timonen, V. (2016) *Beyond Successful and Active Ageing*, Bristol: Policy Press.

Tope, L.G. (2020) 'The role of local authorities in promoting health and wellbeing in the community', in A. Bonner (ed) *Local Authorities and the Social Determinants of Health*, Bristol: Policy Press, pp 83–7.

Tovey, M. (2020) 'Is there a doctor in the house? averting a post-pandemic staffing crisis in the NHS', COVID-19 briefing, Institute of Economic Affairs. Available from: https://iea.org.uk/wp-content/uploads/2020/10/Is-there-a-doctor-in-the-house.pdf

Townsend, P. (1981) 'The structured dependency of the elderly: the creation of social policy in the twentieth century', *Ageing and Society*, 1(1): 5–28.

Toynbee, P. and Walker, D. (2020) *The Lost Decade, 2010–2020 and What Lies Ahead for Britain*, London: Guardian Books.

Tulle, E. (2015) 'Theorising embodiment and ageing', in J. Twigg and W. Martin (eds) *Routledge Handbook of Cultural Gerontology*, London: Routledge, pp 125–32.

Turner, B.S. (1987) *Medical Power and Social Knowledge*, London: SAGE.

Turner, B.S. (2000) 'The history of the changing concepts of health and illness: outline of a general model of illness categories', in G. Albrecht, R. Fitzpatrick, and S. Scrimshaw (eds) *The Handbook of Social Studies in Health and Medicine*, London: SAGE, pp 9–24.

Turner, B.S. (2008) *The Body and Society: Explorations in Social Theory*, New York: City University of New York.

Twigg, J. (2013) *Fashion and Age: Dress, the Body and Later Life*, London: Bloomsbury.

Twigg, J. and Martin, W. (eds) (2015) *Routledge Handbook of Cultural Gerontology*, London: Routledge.

UCU [University and College Union] (2020) 'Universities must not become the care homes of a Covid second wave', 29 August. Available from: https://ucu.org.uk/article/10964/Universities-must-not-become-the-care-homes-of-a-Covid-second-wave

UNISON (2020) 'Care workers put at risk by lack of face masks and basic safety kit, says UNISON: coordinated response needed to protect anxious staff', press release, 31 March. Available from: https://www.unison.org.uk/news/2020/03/care-workers-put-risk-lack-face-masks-basic-safety-kit-says-unison/

Van de Mheen, H.D., Stronks, K. and Mackenback, J.P. (1998) 'A lifecourse perspective on socio-economic inequalities in health: the influence of childhood socio-economic conditions and selection processes', in D. Blane, M. Bartley and G. Davey Smith (eds) *The Sociology of Health Inequalities*, Oxford: Blackwell, pp 193–216.

Volpicelli, G. (2020) 'How Test and Trace failed: England's national contact tracing system is barely functioning. To stop the spread of Covid-19, local authorities are taking matters into their own hands', *WIRED*, 5 November. Available from: https://www.wired.co.uk/article/nhs-test-and-trace-covid-19-failure

Vosko, L. (2010) *Managing the Margins: Gender, Citizenship, and the International Regulation of Precarious Employment*, Oxford: Oxford University Press.

Vosko, L. MacDonald, M. and Campbell, I. (eds) (2009) *Gender and the Contours of Precarious Employment*, London: Routledge.

Wachman, R. (2011) 'Watchdog condemns standards at 28% of Southern Cross homes', *The Guardian*, 12 June. Available from: https://www.theguardian.com/business/2011/jun/12/watchdog-condemns-standards-28-per-cent-southern-cross-homes

Walker, A. (1981) 'Towards a political economy of old age', *Ageing and Society*, 1(1): 73–94.

Walker, A. (2012) 'The new ageism', *The Political Quarterly*, 83(4): 812–19.

Walker, A. and Foster, L. (2013) 'Active ageing: rhetoric, theory and practice', in R. Ervik and T. Skogedal Linden (eds) *The Making of Ageing Policy: Theory and Practice in Europe*, Cheltenham: Edward Elgar, pp 27–52.

Walker, A. and Wong, C.K. (2004) 'The ethnocentric construction of the welfare state', in P. Kennett (ed) *A Handbook of Comparative Social Policy*, Cheltenham and Northampton, MA: Edward Elgar, pp 116–30.

Walker, P., Proctor, K. and Syal, R. (2020) 'Fury as Boris Johnson accuses care homes over high Covid-19 death toll', *The Guardian*, 6 July. Available from: https://www.theguardian.com/society/2020/jul/06/anger-after-johnson-appears-to-blame-care-homes-for-their-high-death-toll

Walsh, M., Stephens, P. and Moore, S. (2000) *Social Policy and Welfare*, Cheltenham: Stanley Thornes.

Walter, T. (2020) *Death in the Modern World*, London: SAGE.

Waring, J. and Bishop, S. (2020) 'Health states of exception: unsafe non-care and the (inadvertent) production of "bare life" in complex care transitions', *Sociology of Health and Illness*, 42(1): 171–90.

Waring, J., Marshall, F. and Bishop, S. (2015) 'Understanding the occupational and organizational boundaries to safe hospital discharge', *Journal of Health Services Research and Policy*, 20(1suppl): 34–44.

WBG [Women's Budget Group] (2020) 'Crises collide: women and Covid-19: examining gender and other equality issues during the Coronavirus outbreak', 9 April. Available from: https://wbg.org.uk/wp-content/uploads/2020/04/FINAL.pdf

Wearden, G. (2011) 'The rise and fall of Southern Cross', *The Guardian*, 1 June. Available from: https://www.theguardian.com/business/2011/jun/01/rise-and-fall-of-southern-cross

Wearing, B. and Wearing, S. (1990) 'Leisure for all? gender policy', in D. Rowe and G. Lawrence (eds) *Sport and Leisure: Trends in Australian Popular Culture*, Sydney, Australia: Harcourt Brace Jovanovich, pp 161–73.

Wearmouth, R. (2020) 'Age UK calls pushing people to sign "do not resuscitate" forms "morally repugnant"', *Huffington Post*, 3 April. Available from: https://www.huffingtonpost.co.uk/entry/do-not-resuscitate-age-uk-coronavirus_uk_5e877643c5b609ebfff0b746?guccounter=1

Webb, E. (2020) 'Coronavirus risk for older people: the updated picture', *Age UK*, 9 June. Available from: https://www.ageuk.org.uk/discover/2020/06/coronavirus-risk-for-older-people-updated/

Wellings, D. (2017) 'The politics of health: what do the public think about the NHS?', The King's Fund, 1 June. Available from: https://www.kingsfund.org.uk/publications/articles/politics-health

White, S. and Hammond, M. (2018) 'From representation to active ageing in a Manchester neighbourhood: fesigning the age-friendly city', in T. Buffel, S. Handler and C. Phillipson (eds) *Age-Friendly Cities and Communities: A Global Perspective*, Bristol: Policy Press, pp 193–210.

Whitfield, D. (2006) *New Labour's Attack on Public Services: Modernisation by Marketisation? How the Commissioning, Choice, Competition and Contestability Agenda Threatens Public Services and the Welfare State*, Nottingham: Spokesman.

WHO [World Health Organization] (2002) 'Active ageing: a policy framework', World Health Organization. Available from: https://extranet.who.int/agefriendlyworld/wp-content/uploads/2014/06/WHO-Active-Ageing-Framework.pdf

Wilson, H. (2017) 'Hands surrenders Four Seasons Health Care to rival H/2 Capital', *The Times*, 9 November. Available from: https://www.thetimes.co.uk/article/hands-surrenders-four-seasons-health-care-to-rival-h-2-capital-rxrv5z87f

Wray, S. (2003) 'Women growing older: ageing, ethnicity and culture', *Sociology*, 37(3): 511–27.

Wray, S. (2004) 'What constitutes agency and empowerment for women in later life?', *The Sociological Review*, 52(1): 22–38.

Wright, J. and Harwood, V. (eds) (2009) *Biopolitics and the 'Obesity Epidemic' Governing Bodies*, Oxfordshire: Routledge.

Wright, O. (2011) 'Care homes operator close to collapse after rents soar', *The Independent*, 15 March. Available from: https://www.independent.co.uk/news/uk/home-news/care-homes-operator-close-to-collapse-after-rents-soar-2241875.html

Wye, L., Lasseter, G., Percival, J., Simmonds, B., Duncan, L. and Purdy, S. (2012) 'Independent evaluation of the Marie Curie Cancer Care Delivering Choice Programme in Somerset and North Somerset', Bristol: Centre for Primary Health Care, Department of Social and Community Medicine, University of Bristol. Available from: https://www.mariecurie.org.uk/globalassets/media/documents/commissioning-our-services/publications/evaluations/dcp-somerset-north-somerset-final-reportpdf

Wye, L., Lasseter, G., Percival, P., Duncan, L., Simmonds, B, Purdy, S. (2014) 'What works in "real life" to facilitate home deaths and fewer hospital admissions for those at end of life? results from a realistic evaluation of new palliative care services in two English counties', *BMC Palliative Care*, 13: 37.

Wye, L., Lasseter, G., Simmonds, B., Duncan, L., Percival, J. and Purdy, S. (2016) 'Electronic palliative care coordinating systems (EPaCCS) may not facilitate home deaths: a mixed methods evaluation of end of life care in two English counties', *Journal of Research in Nursing*, 21(2): 96–107.

Wyman, M.F., Shiovitz-Ezra, S. and Bengel, J. (2018) 'Ageism in the health care system: providers, patients, and systems', in Y. Ayalon and C. Tesch-Romer (eds) *Contemporary Perspectives on Ageism*, New York: Springer Open, pp 193–212.

Yeates, N., Haux, T., Jawad, R. and Kilkey, M. (eds) (2011) *In Defence of Welfare: The Impacts of the Comprehensive Spending Review*, London: Social Policy Association.

Zamora, D. and Behrent, M.C. (2016) (eds) *Foucault and Neoliberalism*, Cambridge: Polity Press.

Zhang, Y.B., Harwood, J., Williams, A., Ylanne-McEwan, V., Wadleigh, P.M. and Thimm, C. (2006) 'The portrayal of older adults in advertising: a cross-national review', *Journal of Language and Social Psychology*, 25(3): 264–82.

Index